Critical

'A very special book filled with stories of survival, hope and loss.'
Adam Kay, author of *This is Going to Hurt: Secret Diaries of a Junior Doctor*

'Matt Morgan is an engaging, honest and perceptive doctor who has managed to pack an awful lot into his career. This book promises to offer a real insight into an area of life-and-death medicine that many of us will have seen dramatised on television.'
Michael Mosley, author of *The Fast 800, The 8-Week Blood Sugar Diet* **and** *The Clever Guts Diet*

'I loved it. So carefully written and obviously as a doctor, I could totally get behind the stories of Gram and the origins of the ICU, but the patients' stories . . . just so touching. I love the exploration of what it means to survive and at what cost.'
Dr Nikki Stamp FRACS, Cardiothoracic and Transplant Surgeon and author of *Can You Die of a Broken Heart? A Heart Surgeon's Insight Into What Makes Us Tick*

'A gripping realism of life in intensive care that reminds us how fragile is life. Written with humility and insight this is an intriguing glimpse into a world of life-saving decisions. It is life affirming and hugely reassuring.'
Professor Dame Sue Black, author of *All That Remains: A Life in Death*

'Matt Morgan writes beautifully and movingly about the edges of life. Through vivid encounters and pitch-perfect insights, he shines a light on the human experience at the frontiers of healthcare.'
Ganesh Suntharalingam, President, Intensive Care Society

'This book is marvellous: buy it, share it, recommend it . . . We are fortunate to have dedicated, caring and humble folks such as Doc Morgan on the critical care front line. We are even better off when a writer can capture all that this exciting, mad, glorious and even exasperating job means. If you work in healthcare, know somebody that does, or simply inhabit a body then this book is for you: in fact it's critical.'
Professor Peter Brindley, Professor of Critical Care Medicine, Anesthesiology, Medical Ethics, University of Alberta

'I am an intensive care doctor and reading *Critical* should have been wholly uninspiring. It was, in fact, quite the reverse. Matt uses language as a great surgeon would a scalpel – with precision, but also grace. I can't commend this book highly enough. My sole regret is that I didn't write it myself.'
Professor Hugh Montgomery

Critical

Science and stories from
the brink of human life

Dr Matt Morgan

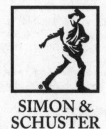

SIMON &
SCHUSTER

London · New York · Sydney · Toronto · New Delhi

A CBS COMPANY

First published in Great Britain by Simon & Schuster UK Ltd, 2019
A CBS COMPANY

Some passages in this book have been adapted from blogs previously published by
The BMJ (British Medical Journal) with permission.

1 3 5 7 9 10 8 6 4 2

Simon & Schuster UK Ltd
1st Floor
222 Gray's Inn Road
London WC1X 8HB

www.simonandschuster.co.uk
www.simonandschuster.com.au
www.simonandschuster.co.in

Simon & Schuster Australia, Sydney
Simon & Schuster India, New Delhi

This book is not intended as a substitute for medical advice or treatment.
Any person with a condition requiring medical attention should
consult a qualified medical practitioner.

The events and clinical scenarios described in this book happened in real life
but some names and other identifying features have, on occasion, been
changed to protect the privacy of colleagues and patients.

Hardback ISBN: 978-1-4711-7303-5
Trade Paperback ISBN: 978-1-4711-8636-3
eBook ISBN: 978-1-4711-7305-9

Typeset in Bembo by M Rules
Printed and bound in Australia by Griffin Press

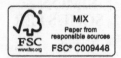

MIX
Paper from
responsible sources
FSC
www.fsc.org FSC® C009448

For my mum and dad,
who taught me that anything is possible

Author's Note

I have changed some of the personal details of patients in order to help protect their privacy. Where cases are likely to disclose a patient's identity through their unusual nature, I have sought patient consent – or assent from their relatives – to share these details with the reader. While all clinical cases are based on real patients I have met, I have combined some of their stories and improved the narrative for the reader. I have only included facts that I believe to be true, although I have not sought independent verification of second-hand details given to me by colleagues, families or friends. Some of the themes discussed in this book have been adapted and expanded upon from my blogs published by The BMJ (British Medical Journal).

CONTENTS

PREFACE

In 2016, I attended a medical conference in Dublin, Ireland. The speakers were brilliant, the venue impressive and the whole experience inspiring. On the final day, I left with a real sense of hope and motivation, eager to face my day job as an intensive care consultant, fizzing with new ideas. That evening, serendipity took me by the hand to an old Irish bar and changed my life. A local asked me what I was doing in the city. I explained that I had been at a medical conference.

'Oh great,' she said. 'What kind of doctor are you?'

'I'm an intensivist,' I replied.

'What on earth is that?' she asked.

At that moment, something profound struck me. I had spent the last decade writing academic research papers that few people would ever read. I had travelled the world, speaking at medical conferences to audiences who understood the topics that I spoke about better than I. Despite all of this hard work and effort, I'd forgotten about the most important person: you.

You are my past patient, my future patient, the son, daughter, father, mother or neighbour of my current patient. Although one in five of you admitted will eventually die in an intensive care unit, many of you won't even know what that is.

That cold Irish evening, through the dark mist of my final Guinness, I started writing this book. It is not a book filled with joy – indeed, there will be sadness – but there is always hope. I will take you on a journey to the light and the dark places that critically ill patients visit. Even in death, glimmers of the future can reflect in the smallest of spaces. I will borrow the bodies, the lives and the families of real patients I have met, and I will use them to shed light into these deep cracks where life meets death.

If I work hard today, tomorrow and the day after that, I may save one life. In my whole career, I may save hundreds. However, I hope this book will achieve far more. I hope that it will show you what intensive care can, should and perhaps should not do. It will offer you powerful insights that may prevent those close to you from ever needing to meet me. It will even teach you how to save a life. It will raise your awareness of the most significant harms in society and allow you to glimpse at the very edges of life. The fragility of life will become clear, yet this will be shown to be offset by the incredible resilience and tenacity of humanity.

I will now take you on a journey through the world of intensive care, offering you a glimpse of the patients we treat every day, with each chapter inspired by the people

I have met at the front line of clinical medicine. We will explore the inner workings of the physical ICU (intensive care unit) as well as my mind as a doctor working within it. You will experience the sounds, smells and sights of the most dramatic area of the hospital. We will travel through the main organ systems of the human body, find out how we can keep people alive without a pulse, and what happens when a patient becomes brainstem dead. I will share with you the highs and the lows that patients, families and healthcare staff witness through the course of fighting human fragility. While the lows can be dark, I am privileged to support patients and their families while they stand at the brink of existence. Through this lens, I am reminded daily of the beauty of life. The late Steve Jobs said in a Stanford commencement address that 'death was life's greatest invention', allowing us to appreciate the time we have on this earth to share with others. Sometimes darkness can show you the light.

Dr Matt Morgan
@dr_mattmorgan
January 2019

1

An Introduction to the World of Intensive Care Medicine

How a little girl helped to save the world

```
Intensive care doctor:
intensivist, critical care doctor,
intensive care medicine doctor,
resuscitationist, but, ultimately,
just a human.
```

It was a beautiful sunny August evening in Copenhagen as Vivi danced in her garden after returning home from school. She was a happy twelve-year-old girl, with sandy-golden hair and apple-red cheeks. Life was tough since her parents had separated; her mum struggled to make ends meet working as a hatmaker. She watched her daughter through the window, dancing barefoot on the grass as she giggled and smiled to herself. Forty-eight hours later, Vivi was about to die. This is the story of the people, practices and technology which allowed her instead to live. Her journey was the first step along a sixty-five-year-long journey that now enables us to enjoy life in the face of devastating critical illness. This is the story of how intensive care can save your life.

Vivi didn't notice the moment earlier that day when a water droplet landed on her hand.* Nor did she know that a million copies of the deadly poliomyelitis virus were in that water droplet as she rubbed her eyes at night. As her mother's lullaby sent her to sleep, the virus started its work. It travelled from her hands to the cells in her mouth, before passing through the cell membranes. As the sun went down, the virus infected her tonsils, the lymph nodes in her neck and finally her intestines. By the morning Vivi had a head-ache which stopped her from dancing. Her mum's cool hand felt Vivi's hot head and rubbed her stiff neck. The next day Vivi struggled to fasten the buttons on her summer dress. Her fingers moved clumsily at the end of two heavy, weak arms. After being taken to the local Blegdam Hospital, she stopped responding to her name, as her breathing became rapid and shallow. Soon Vivi met the man who would save her life. He was the world's first intensive care doctor, Dr Bjorn Ibsen (Appendix: Figure 1).

Dr Ibsen was a 36-year-old anaesthetist when he met

---

* While transmission via water particles was most likely and typical for this infection, it is impossible to say with certainty that this is the exact path of transmission in Vivi's case.

Vivi. It was clear to him that she was suffering from acute severe polio (acute meaning the disease started and progressed rapidly; severe because Vivi's polio caused her profound weakness). Twenty-seven people had already died of the disease in just the first two weeks of the Copenhagen polio outbreak in 1952. Before its end, more than three hundred people would contract polio, a third with the severe respiratory failure that Vivi was developing, with 130 people dying as a result. Dr Ibsen knew that the so-called iron lung – the last machine that could save Vivi – was already in use. This machine was Vivi's only chance of surviving the illness that had caused her respiratory muscles to become too weak to turn the air around her into breath. The iron lung created an airtight seal between a patient's chest and the outside world, allowing a powerful air pump to make a vacuum that would suck out the chest wall and cause air to flow into the lungs through the windpipe.

Dr Ibsen felt helpless as he watched Vivi's breathing become even shallower. The build-up of dissolved carbon dioxide gas in her bloodstream, normally removed by breathing, pushed her blood pressure ever higher and depressed her consciousness so much that she could no longer stop her saliva from choking her. Dr Ibsen decided to do something radical that would change medicine for ever.

In an operating theatre, Dr Ibsen's job as an anaesthetist was to administer powerful drugs that would render a person unconscious and then to use other drugs to stop all muscle contractions, including those of the breathing muscles. Only under these circumstances could a surgeon safely perform complex operations that required still and controlled access to the inside of the human body. To keep a patient alive in the meantime, Dr Ibsen would need to breathe for his patients by inserting a plastic tube into the trachea, or windpipe. Although normally inserted through the mouth or nose, occasionally a tube would be inserted directly into the trachea through the front of the neck – a procedure known as a tracheotomy.

For Dr Ibsen, Vivi's condition mirrored that of the patients he cared for every day. The difference here was that the muscle weakness was caused by the polio virus acting directly on the motor nerves and spinal cord that normally supplied Vivi's muscles with instructions. However, the solution was the same, and at 11.15 a.m. on 27 August 1952 Dr Ibsen took Vivi to the operating theatre, organised an emergency tracheotomy, attached the pipe in her trachea to an inflatable bag that he then squeezed, forcing air into the lungs using positive pressure.

This is the opposite of how humans normally breathe. Take a deep breath in right now and feel the large muscle in your abdomen, your diaphragm, pushing down while simultaneously the muscles between your ribs contract, pulling them upwards and outwards. Together this creates a negative pressure in the layers between the elastic lungs and the inside of the ribcage. This pressure is transmitted to the lungs, pulling them outwards, dropping the pressure in the 500 million tiny air sacs inside, and thus drawing in air. This is the moment when air becomes breath. Instead, though, Dr Ibsen was squeezing a bag to push air into the lungs, much like what happens if you hang your head out of a fast-moving car's window and open your mouth.

After one breath, Vivi's chest went up and then down. The second breath was easier than the first, and by the tenth breath her heavy eyes opened and she saw through life's windows once again.

It is often the simple ideas in life that lead to the most profound change. This was one such moment. To sustain and not just save a life, Dr Ibsen needed to take the next important step – to create a safe place in which to keep Vivi and gather a team of people to care for her by squeezing the bag until her respiratory muscles had recovered. No one knew how long this might take. In fact it took a team of medical students working shifts of up to eight hours each, continuously squeezing the bag – not too hard, not too softly – for months in a small temporary hospital ward to keep Vivi alive (Appendix: Figure 2). This was the world's first intensive care unit, requiring over 1,500 volunteer medical students to squeeze Vivi's bag and then the bags of countless other patients day in, day out for six months during the Copenhagen polio epidemic. Finally, in January 1953, the bag was replaced with a dedicated mechanical ventilator that would breathe for Vivi.

Against the odds, and despite being unable to move from the neck downwards, Vivi survived. Seven long years after becoming ill, she left hospital and moved into a newly built apartment complex with her mother that allowed her to live attached to her breathing machine twenty-four hours a day. Vivi was an extremely happy, lively and brave young lady. She had a passion for reading, using a stick in her mouth to turn the pages of her favourite books (Appendix: Figure 3), and she would paint jewellery by using a paintbrush held between her teeth. She often travelled to family parties, always accompanied by heavy batteries strapped underneath her wheelchair to power her mechanical lungs, and her beloved Border collie, Bobby, would help her pass the time while looking over the skyline of Copenhagen from the twelfth-floor apartment block. In time Vivi formed a special bond with one of her male carers, and the pair fell in love and were soon engaged, finding respite from the reality of Vivi's situation by spending long summer days together at a family summer house along with her dog Bobby.

Despite Vivi's years of extensive rehabilitation and care, the ongoing burden of disability that often accompanies survival from critical illness prevented her from regaining her full independence. Yet Vivi did not let the challenges she faced cast a shadow over what she had been gifted. Her mum had her daughter back, Vivi had her life back, and Dr Ibsen never looked back. Nor would medicine.

~

Intensive care is not simply a place, a collection of people or a life-support machine. Like a modern-day church, it uses specially designed buildings, expensive equipment, particular methods, and people trained in the art and practices of a certain tradition to focus all of their attention on one thing. Rather than the immortal god, intensive care focuses on the very mortal patient, caring for the sickest patient in any hospital.

The physical location can be called the intensive care unit (ICU), the high-dependency unit or simply critical care. It should contain 10 per cent of the total number of beds in the hospital and be located close to the operating theatres and the emergency department. Each individual bed area has specialised equipment including a life-support or breathing machine, multiple medication pumps, dialysis machines and monitoring equipment. The most important item next to each bed, however, is none of these. It is a patient's own nurse.

All patients in intensive care are there because they have failure of one or more of their vital organs. This could be lung failure, requiring a breathing machine as in the case of Vivi, but also heart failure, kidney failure, gut failure, metabolic failure, blood failure or even brain failure. Anyone with this degree of illness, requiring organ support, is critically ill. We can classify the severity of a patient's illness throughout the hospital – and the subsequent care that they need – into five different levels from 0 to 4. Level 0 patients are those with a relatively mild illness that can be safely treated in a normal hospital ward with one nurse per seven to twenty patients. Level 1 patients are those at risk of deterioration, who require more regular observations of their vital signs. They will often be cared for in an acute ward setting, with more frequent nursing interventions. Level 2 is where high-dependency care is needed. These patients are people with only one organ failing and they will be nursed in a ratio of one nurse to two patients. This is often delivered in an area that is next to, or even includes, intensive care. Meanwhile, sicker patients require level 3 care, where a highly trained nurse will be at their bedside every hour of every day. This most often occurs when patients need a life-support machine to help them breathe or where more than one organ system is failing. Occasionally, a patient needs so much complex equipment that they require more than one nurse. These patients are termed level 4 and they are always treated in an ICU. Here critically ill patients require not only special medicines or machines, but also time: time to dedicate care to their problems, and equipment to allow time for their bodies to heal. Essential to all of this is the dedicated nursing time they are given.

The skills an intensive care doctor needs are broad. We perform surgery by inserting tubes into people's chests, necks and blood vessels. We must be expert communicators, often meeting families for the first time to tell them the worst news of their lives. We help perform and interpret medical scans of every body part, from X-rays of bones to CT scans of the brain. We adjust the physiology of the body with powerful drugs that we must know like the back of our hands. Our environment is covered in monitors, displaying hundreds of pieces of information, glowing with complex, multi-coloured waveforms. We combine all of these skills to work out what is wrong with someone as their body struggles to live. We then try to fix the problems we have found by co-ordinating a team of people who can help.

Sometimes the breadth of knowledge and skills needed make me feel like an imposter in my own hospital. The first time I felt like this was in 2003. I was a medical student presenting to a large, polished audience of esteemed military plastic surgeons during their annual meeting. After spending a summer training in the Nevada desert with American military doctors, I wanted to share my experiences of this simulated battlefield exercise. As I stood up, the projector bulb flashing to life, my voice froze. For what seemed like an eternity, I just looked out at the perfectly ironed audience, asking myself: 'What right do I have to be here?' In some ways I was right to doubt myself: I was barely qualified to talk on this topic to an audience overflowing with experience. Fortunately, something clicked as my first slide hung on the projector screen behind me and the next twenty minutes flew past, but in the officers' mess afterwards, when people told me how much they had enjoyed my talk, I did not believe them.

Fifteen years later, I am perfectly qualified to speak on many subjects, but when I present at a medical conference, these feelings sometimes return, as they do for many other doctors. It is no wonder that we intensive care doctors feel unsure of ourselves when expected to assimilate the 13,000 diagnoses, 6,000 drugs and 4,000 surgical procedures that we may need in order to treat almost any disease at any time. It feels like being a family doctor, expected to know the entirety of medicine, except applying it only to the sickest patients. Our skills of being able to ask the right questions and knowing where to find the answers trumps any rote-learnt medical knowledge. In the hospital, we often barge into other medical specialities at a moment's notice, treating conditions that we may not have encountered for years, before leaving as swiftly as we arrived. We are expert problem-solvers, thinking on our feet while trying to keep our brain based on evidence.

Many of the notable moments in my career have involved this type of problem-solving rather than the recall of bland medical facts. While working in an emergency department, I remember thirty-two muddied rugby players from the local under-10s team squeezing into a busy waiting room one Saturday afternoon. A practical joke played by one of the opposing players – adding menthol muscle rub to the after-match curry – had backfired. All thirty-two children were holding bottles of water, constantly washing out their burning, minty mouths. After checking the chemical content of the muscle rub, it transpired a hot tongue was the least of their worries. The cream contained aspirin as the active ingredient, the willow-bark extract originally used by ancient Egyptians as a remedy for aches and pains. Unfortunately, aspirin is also a toxic drug when used in excess quantities, especially by children. Now faced with a waiting room full of scared children and worried parents, the standard approach of testing blood levels in every individual was less than ideal due to the time it would take. A more creative medical problem-solving approach was needed, so I stood at the entrance of the waiting room, the air thick with the smell of dirty boots and mud, and loudly asked: 'WHICH ONE OF YOU ATE THE MOST CURRY?'

Thankfully, a slim, young boy put up his hand, remembering how his friends had laughed at him for finishing his meal so quickly before his taste buds had been awoken by the menthol. We took him to one side and tested his blood. I read the results with relief, seeing that the level of salicylate acid (the chemical name for aspirin) was well below the threshold needing treatment. We could safely assume, given the boy's big appetite and his low weight compared with his peers, that the remaining players could all return to the pitch. There could only be one person deserving of man of the match after his blood test had spared his teammates from the sharp end of a needle.

~

When posed a tricky question during my post-graduate examinations, I would often play for time by responding with my stock phrase: 'Well, let's divide this answer into three main parts ...' The few extra seconds this response gave me would bump-start my brain into generating at least one out of the three answers I had promised. However, when answering the question 'How do patients get into the

ICU?', there genuinely are three possible answers: the front door, the side door or the theatre door.

The emergency department is colloquially known as the hospital's 'front door'. It is the main route of entry for patients arriving by road or air ambulance, for patients self-presenting in an emergency or even for patients rolled out from a speeding car as I once witnessed. Those whose measurements of their physiological signs – including heart rate, blood pressure and conscious state – lead to them being assessed as critically ill are taken directly to an area called 'resus' in the emergency department. Short for 'resuscitation', this zone has individual patient bays ideally set up to care for the sickest of patients in an efficient, timely manner. Each area in resus has emergency drugs on stand-by, equipment to put you onto a life-support machine close at hand, and a high ratio of staff all trained and ready to save your life. It is like a miniature ICU that needs to act fast but only for a short period of time. Some doctors specialise in treating patients at this stage of their journey and call themselves resuscitationists. Intensive care doctors will visit resus when critically ill patients are referred to them.

As an intensive care consultant, there are some instantly recognisable numbers that flash up on my battered mobile pager time after time. Just reading the digits 915 – the number for resus – gives my adrenal gland a call to action even when I am sitting safely in my local pub ten miles away from the hospital. Resus is often the most exciting and dangerous point to care for patients as they arrive from the tangled outside world, covered in dirt, blood and jeans and with little prior information to go on. If you panic, they panic and others panic – and panic has never saved a life. As I walk through the red doors, never knowing what will be ahead, I mentally rehearse my most feared scenarios, take a slow deep breath and form an external veneer of calm to temper the maelstrom inside. I try to make pools of order in a sea of disorder. Intensivists often help to stabilise patients during this early phase of their illness, assisting in making a diagnosis or short-term plans as well as deciding whether patients are suitable for admission to the ICU. Only when the seas are calm are patients then safe to move on to the next stage of their journey to our ICU if they remain critically ill.

Around one-third of my patients are admitted to intensive care directly from another hospital ward – via the 'side door'. They may have spent days, weeks or even months in hospital before becoming ill enough to need critical care. The challenge in caring for a ward patient is very different compared with the blank slate of a resus patient. Stepping onto an unfamiliar ward to see a referral, I have a secret technique to quickly find the critically ill patient. Scanning the area, a curtain will be drawn around one bed space, with the feet of multiple nurses and doctors just visible under the bottom edge of this cloth barrier. Some feet stand still, watching. Others frantically move around this way and then that way. As I approach, the familiar beep of hospital monitors will be heard. Peering around the curtain, the details I have been told by the referring team merge with the image before me to form my immediate gut instinct.

Ward patient referrals come with a wealth of information, multiple test results, X-rays, pages of notes and – most dangerously – the opinions of others. Most errors in clinical reasoning are not due to incompetence or poor knowledge but are intrinsic to the software of human thinking. When confronted with time pressures, large amounts of data, complexity and uncertainty, our brain takes several reasonable shortcuts. It uses heuristics to short-circuit the need for deep thinking and instead relies upon experience, the opinions of others and decisions that reassure us. When our ancient ancestors were faced with a herd of wildebeest on the hot savannah, these shortcuts saved their lives; when we are faced with a critically ill patient on the ward, these shortcuts may save far fewer.

Today, when I am told by a colleague that, for example, a patient on the trauma ward is short of breath three days after a car accident due to severe infection, my instinct is to believe this. I look at their blood results, subconsciously focusing on those that confirm the assumption I have already made. I remember the face of the last patient I admitted from that same ward who died due to severe infection and I become determined that this time things will be different. My ape brain is happy, but my critical thinking is not. I cannot allow these shortcuts to be the end of my process. I need insight and training to warn me about these shortcuts that my other self is making. I need to go back to the start, to think for myself, be logical, and ask: 'What if that *isn't* the problem?' If I do not do this, I will miss the fact that this latest patient does not have an infection at all and that, in fact, they are bleeding inside – profusely, non-stop. Antibiotics and a life-support machine certainly would not help. What this latest patient needs is a surgeon to stop their bleeding. Thankfully the development of critical care as a specialty comes with insights from cognitive science, addressing some defects inherent to the human condition.

I have made a lot of mistakes as a doctor. However, I am not a bad doctor. What I am is a normal human, working in an abnormal environment. Most mistakes made in medicine relate not to deficits in knowledge or skill. I used to worry about missing that rare diagnosis or making complex procedural errors at the worst time, but I have never done this. I now know that the mistakes I have made – and am likely to make in the future – will be simple, predictable errors, not complex ones. They are the types of blunder that you will make tomorrow while shopping, talking with friends or driving. The conclusions we leap to based on heuristics often are correct, but they can also be wrong. You will search in the same place three times while looking for your house keys, convinced you left them right there. You will visit the shops and forget the one item that you went there for in the first place. But life will carry on.

Sadly, when a patient is balanced on the edges of life, these simple errors can lead to disaster. These are tolerated in other industries such as accountancy, banking or software development. In medicine, they can result in pain, suffering or death. Yet the same humans are involved.

The recognition of medical error as human error has allowed a gradual transformation in healthcare systems. Today it should be possible for a doctor to make a potentially serious mistake and for the system to prevent this from harming a patient. I may try to inject a fatal amount of air through a tube into a vein instead of the stomach, but a special attachment will prevent me from being able to do so. Intensive care nurtures a robust system that should be able to fail gracefully not catastrophically. It should compensate, have resilience and redundancy, in anticipation of human error. However, it is in no way perfect and has a long way to go.

These improvements have been achieved through three strands of innovation. Atul Gawande's paradigm-shifting book, *The Checklist Manifesto*, introduced to medicine simple yet effective techniques you already use when shopping to remember those essential items. His introduction of the World Health Organization's 'Surgical Safety Checklist' has saved millions of lives by ensuring that simple critical steps, such as checking a patient's name and allergies, are carried out for each and every operation. We have now adapted his checklists for intensive care procedures such as tracheotomies and daily ward rounds.

The second strand has borrowed techniques used in industries such as aviation to allow improved team behaviour during a crisis. Crew resource management (CRM) empowers junior staff to question the decisions made by senior members of the team, flattening hierarchy and thereby improving safety. CRM can help teams come together in the fog of a disaster and work together effectively and safely. During emergencies in critical care, I now take a step backwards rather than forwards to get an overview of the situation, assign roles and act on good ideas provided by others.

The final transformative strand was built on the work of Nobel Prize-winning Daniel Kahneman in his life-affirming book, *Thinking, Fast and Slow*. Recognising that medical error is effectively a manifestation of ingrained human heuristics has allowed commonly described cognitive errors to be anticipated in healthcare. Every day, I see evidence of anchoring bias, where an incorrect diagnostic label is permanently attached to a patient after being applied earlier by another doctor. I am aware I often test patients for rare diagnoses in the days after I care for another patient with that very diagnosis. I know that I seek information to confirm my gut feelings, often disposing of inconvenient facts that would otherwise produce psychological conflict known as cognitive dissonance. Mentally preparing myself for these human bugs can stop them from becoming ends in themselves. Knowing about them makes me a better intensive care doctor.

The final route of entry to the ICU – via the 'theatre door' – is for selected post-surgery patients. This can be in a planned manner or as the result of complications arising from the operation or anaesthesia. Certain major operations will need a period of heightened observation or organ support when the surgery is finished. These operations include major cancer surgery to the oesophagus, removing parts of a diseased lung, and heart operations. Sometimes, though an operation may not be a major procedure, the background ill health of the patient will necessitate admission to intensive care in a planned manner. Predicting this is difficult. Some hospitals offer exercise testing to analyse a patient's ability to cope with an operation. These tests are time-consuming, costly and not all patients can manage them. The explosion of consumer wearable technology prompted me to question whether simply wearing a watch measuring physiological signs could act as a surrogate for these more invasive tests. Although our research is ongoing, perhaps in the next ten years, wearable technology will improve our risk-prediction models to better care for patients after major surgery.

The planned need for post-surgery ICU admissions leads to significant challenges. Aside from the regular surges that can be anticipated throughout the winter, the capacity of a critical care unit is difficult to predict on a daily basis. Therefore, if your operation requires an intensive care bed, your fate can be determined by the busyness of the hospital the night prior to your operation. When faced with a critically ill patient who needs that last intensive care bed following a car accident, what would you tell the patient needing that bed to have their cancer surgery the next morning? There are only a limited number of times that surgeons, intensivists and nurses can say sorry to a patient before it sounds hollow. All too often the outcome from this pressurised system, running at nearly 100 per cent capacity, is that operations are frequently postponed. Although capacity expansion is the most obvious solution, it comes with significant financial costs. Therefore, the drive for healthcare efficiency has led to other solutions being explored. Any capacity in the system is seen as slack by finance departments rather than as an essential part of patient safety. Without the ability to flex, the system is stiff and fragile with a tendency to snap.

One innovative solution involves having an area of intensive care with absolutely no beds. This seems like a strange way to solve the issue of not having an empty bed, but often the lack of an available intensive care bed is because patients who have improved in the ICU do not then have a standard ward bed to move on to. Instead, having only a physical space in intensive care allows a patient to be admitted to an elective surgical ward, have their operation and then come to critical care on that same physical ward bed they arrived in. After twenty-four hours of close observation, they can then return to the same physical space on the ward where they were first admitted, and the cycle can then continue. This simple yet effective strategy has allowed hundreds of operations to proceed in the last year where previously many may have been cancelled.

～

Sixty-five years after that long hot summer in Copenhagen, the ICU is a very different place. Nearly every emergency hospital in the Western world now has a dedicated area, specially designed to look after critically ill patients. We no longer need the shifts of medical students who were used as breathing machines to keep patients alive during the polio epidemic in Copenhagen in 1952. Today, intensive care stands at the cutting edge of medicine, both technologically and through our use of highly specialised staff, drugs and therapies. This all involves significant costs, with a single night spent in intensive care costing as much as £3,000. As well as these financial costs, the human resource challenges required to look after patients are huge. A typical critical care team consists of one-to-one nursing, healthcare assistants, a team of general and specialist doctors, a pharmacist, a physiotherapist, a dietician, an occupational therapist, a social worker, a psychologist and a host of support services. Despite concerns about the high cost of intensive care treatments, it has been shown that treating a patient in ICU is cheaper than many other therapies including drugs used in primary-care settings. For example, analysis suggests that the cost for each additional life saved in intensive care is around £40,000, compared with £220,000 for the treatment of high cholesterol using statins in well patients.

Treating the most critically ill patients in ICU can markedly reduce their chances of dying. The average mortality rate for these patients has been incrementally decreasing over time thanks to better systems, better training, better equipment and evidence-based therapies. There are now more than 30 million patients admitted to intensive care worldwide every year, of whom 24 million people will survive. We can therefore estimate that, since Vivi became its first patient, intensive care has resulted in around half a billion people surviving critical illness. Yet it is not just maintaining life that has been an aim for critical care. When I look into a mother's eyes and tell her that we will do all we can to save her son, I mean that we will strive to save the quality of life that her son had before he was unwell. Evidence shows that intensive care is able to significantly increase the chance of survival from critical illness and of leading a meaningful life, not just being alive.

~

In the twenty years after becoming the first intensive care patient in the world, Vivi had grown up, fallen in love, got engaged and read endless books. Life was filled with colour and laughter. Sadly, however, as Vivi turned thirty, she became seriously ill. Her lungs remained weak, her breathing shallow, and she returned to Blegdam Hospital – this time not with polio, but as a consequence of escaping death the first time. Her shallow breathing meant she had recurrent chest infections, but this one was different. She was admitted in September 1971 with pneumonia, and this time she would not go home. She died peacefully, aged just thirty-two. Intensive care had given her a second chance at life twenty years earlier but it could not save her now.

Indeed, sixty-seven years later, it still cannot save everyone and we still have a lot to learn. We need to find out how being in intensive care can affect patients years after they have recovered. We need to debate the ethical and moral questions surrounding who *should* be treated and not only who *can* be treated. We need to develop as a specialty so that, if Vivi were brought into my hospital that second time today, she would not die. We also need to show the public what is possible, what is right, and what is not.

2

THE IMMUNE SYSTEM

Gatekeeper, defender, traitor and attacker

Christopher was a seventeen-year-old student with the world at his feet. Passionate about travel, he counted the days until his school trip to Australia before starting at university. In a last-minute change of heart, he opted instead to join his friend visiting Kenya. It would be a decision that altered the lives of his friends and family for ever. It would also change my life.

Christopher's dad was never comfortable with this sudden change of plan. He didn't want his son to go to Africa. He tied a piece of red wool to Christopher's new backpack and another to the roof of the car as they left for the airport. He told his wife that he would only untie that red wool when Christopher had returned home safely.

The voluntary work with children in the local African slum was just what Christopher had been hoping for. It allowed him to become immersed in the daily lives of others, experiencing life through a very different lens from what he was accustomed to. Two weeks into his trip, Christopher joined some friends on a hike to the summit of Mount Kenya, his strong lungs and powerful limbs allowing him to help an older lady to make the climb. Some of the local children he had befriended joined him for a triumphant photo at the summit (Appendix: Figure 4). They later swam together in a hotel pool after making the descent in the shadow of the mountain known as the roof of Africa. That night as he slept, baboons would drink the pool water in which Christopher swam, as they had done on countless occasions before.

The next day, Christopher developed symptoms of a cold, with a temperature and a dry cough. These were the early stages of an infection that had possibly invaded his body during the swim that felt so good at the time. Any break in the barriers that normally keep foreign intruders out, such as a minor skin cut, can lead to microorganisms entering your body. These can include viruses, bacteria, fungi and even protozoa. Due to the way in which the human breathing system is arranged – with millions of the lungs' tiny air sacs in constant close contact with the dirty air outside and the bloodstream on the inside – the lungs are by far the most common site of infection. Other routes of entry into the body include the urinary system, through a break in the wall of the bowel, across the bowel wall itself or through body cavities such as the air-filled nasal sinuses.

Christopher decided to take it easy the following day

while his friends ventured further into the mountain range. By mid-afternoon, he was short of breath and coughing up thick green sputum. By the evening he was struggling to breathe and vomiting. He was taken to a local clinic, where doctors found evidence of a chest infection. Touch your forehead now and you will feel the near-constant temperature of 37°C maintained within a fraction of a degree, even on the hottest or coldest day of the year. Count the number of times you are breathing per minute: it should be between ten and fifteen. Instead, Christopher had a high temperature of over 39°C, an elevated heart rate of over 120 beats per minute and a rapid rate of breathing of over twenty-five times per minute. There were crackles at the bottom of his right lung, resulting from fluid filling the delicate air sacs. At the local hospital, an X-ray of Christopher's chest showed fluffy white areas where the black appearance of air should have been. Termed *consolidation*, this is how infection appears on an X-ray. Christopher had pneumonia.

Any form of life can cause human infections. Globally, parasites and helminths (worms) are a significant source of human suffering. In the Western world, it is viruses and bacteria, followed by fungi, that lead to the most problems. A hundred thousand viruses can fit onto the surface of a pinhead, the smallest being just 20 nanometres across, although that number is far less at 5,000 for the smallest bacteria and just 500 for fungi. These are all tiny yet very much alive and can lead to pain, suffering and death, even for an organism as complex and evolutionarily adapted as a human being.

Severe infections that cause multi-organ failure are most commonly caused by bacteria. These bacteria can be divided into two neat groups according to the chemicals used to form their outer cell wall barrier. In 1882, the Danish scientist Hans Christian Gram added a crystal violet dye to a group of bacteria. They took up the purple colour in their outer wall and were subsequently termed 'Gram-positive'. Those that did not take up this stain were called 'Gram-negative'. This simple classification system has allowed scientists to draw a family tree for different microbe types according to whether they take up the Gram stain, the way that they look microscopically and how they group together. Those that collect into a string-of-beads pattern and take up the Gram stain, for example, are termed *Streptococcus*, while those found in clusters are known as *Staphylococcus*. Knowing what type of bug is causing infection gives clues about where an illness may have originated (such as from the lungs as opposed to the brain) and guides our choice of antibiotics. Christopher had an infection with the string-like bacteria, *Streptococcus*, likely contracted from his swim in that pool in Africa.

Christopher was given antibiotics into his veins, the treatment shown to be most effective in severe infection, yet he deteriorated. His breathing became faster and shallower as he became tired. The tiny air sacs in his lungs, which normally allowed the 21 per cent of oxygen in the air to travel across a layer 200 times thinner than a human hair and into the bloodstream, became filled with infected waste. This first affected his body's ability to take up oxygen from the air and then his ability to remove the waste carbon dioxide gas through his lungs. As the carbon dioxide level increased in his blood, Christopher became drowsy and fell unconscious. A plastic tube was inserted, the thickness of your middle finger, into his mouth between his vocal cords and into his windpipe. Using drugs to stop his muscles from contracting, this process is called tracheal intubation. The tube has a soft inflatable balloon around the edges to make a watertight seal between the upper airway and the lungs. He was put onto a life-support machine that blew air with ever-increasing amounts of oxygen into his lungs, while passively letting exhaled breath containing carbon dioxide leave. Christopher had developed sepsis – an overwhelming immune response of his body to infection, causing tissue damage and organ failure.

The time that I spent with Christopher after he was transferred by plane to our intensive care unit in the UK radically altered the path I followed through my medical career, and for that I am very grateful. Rather than continuing along the route to become an intensive care specialist, I paused my clinical training to complete a research PhD, attempting to answer the questions that I found myself asking in the wake of Christopher's illness. For three years, I would take blood samples from critically ill patients in the early stages of severe infection known as sepsis, and use lasers, dyes, enzymes and microscopes to look at the building blocks of their immune system. I quickly discovered that sepsis, the Latin term meaning 'to rot', is a devastating, complex disease where patients need their body to respond in just the right way in order to survive. Too much of an immune reaction and they risk multi-organ failure like Christopher; too little and life can quickly fizzle out without a fight. They need to be like Goldilocks with her porridge: the immune response should be not too hot, yet not too cold, just right.

Once a microbe gains entry to the body, it has a fight on its hands. From infancy, white blood cells – first identified by Dr William Hewson, a British country doctor, in 1774 – constantly roam around inside us, getting acquainted with and memorising all the parts that normally constitute our body, and hoping to recognise intruders that do not belong. Some parts of a bacteria, for example, are made from substances not normally found inside the human body, and immune cells recognise these 'non-self' substances – such as the outer coating of the bacteria that had infected Christopher's lungs.

Next follows a process that is responsible for both the effectiveness of the immune system and also its dangers – cascade and amplification. This is a bit like a snowball rolling down a steep mountain. The immune cells activated by these 'non-self' substances call for help with simple hormone messages that attract a range of other cells to flood the area, arriving like a snowball – faster and faster, bigger and bigger – via blood vessels that have become floppy and wide due to the action of secreted nitric oxide. In other diseases, including severe lung failure, we add nitric oxide to the air patients breathe to exploit this gas's property of relaxing blood vessels. These newly arriving cells include those that can entirely engulf the trespassers and unleash vast amounts of strong 'bleach', protein bullets that shoot through the bacteria walls, and even substances that hijack the DNA blueprints of the bacteria, causing them to attack themselves and die.

Other immune cells arrive, called T-cells after their development early in life from the thymus gland in the neck. Like an experienced police officer on the beat, they may have met the same trespassers before. If so, they release vast amounts of protein antibodies that destroy the bacteria and call yet more officers to help in the battle, continuing the process of cascade and amplification like an ever-growing chemical snowball.

Yet more cells then flood out of the lymphatic system, travelling throughout the body at speeds of more than half a metre per hour, navigating along the inside surface of tissues by sniffing out minuscule signals released from infected cells like police sniffer dogs. We become aware of this process when we develop a temperature caused by the hormones released, notice swelling of the infected parts of our body due to blood vessel engorgement, and become tired due to the sheer energy needed for this police chase. The immune system will hopefully resolve the situation, clearing the infection so that we recover, ready to face another day.

Sadly, this doesn't always happen. In Christopher's case,

the reactions that his body used to clear the infection had a number of unwanted and serious side effects. Multi-organ failure can occur after serious infections and, rarely, even after minor ones. The question is, why does this happen? There are three critical determinants: the bug, the person and the treatment. We will examine each in turn after returning to Christopher.

By now, Christopher's heart had become affected by his illness. The millions of *Streptococcus* bacteria responsible for his infection were starting to die as the powerful antibiotics blasted holes in the surface of their cells. But the chain reaction that had already started meant that this came too late. Christopher's body was reacting so forcefully to try to destroy the bacteria that it was affecting the health of his organs. His blood pressure dropped too low for blood to flow effectively to his brain and to his kidneys. In an attempt to compensate, Christopher's heart rate increased from around a healthy sixty beats per minute to over 140 beats per minute. He had developed shock.

His blood-clotting system also reacted to the bacteria, his blood becoming thick and prone to clumping, which blocked the tiny vessels supplying his fingers, toes and kidneys. As a result, his hands became cold, his fingers pale and his kidneys were no longer able to remove the waste materials produced by his body. At the same time, his blood was too thin in other areas, causing bleeding around the tubes placed into his blood vessels. The fluid that the doctors were pouring into Christopher's veins to increase his blood pressure now leaked out between the lining of his blood vessels, as his body's reaction to the infection destroyed the normally tight seals between these different compartments. Christopher had developed multi-organ failure because of sepsis. We had used the techniques of both Gram and Koch from distant history to successfully identify the bug causing this as *Streptococcus pneumoniae*.

It has been 140 years since the discovery of the germ theory by the German scientist Robert Koch. He was the first to robustly show that infection was transmitted by tiny, invisible microorganisms rather than alternative means, including 'bad air'. The development of optical microscopes helped in this revolution, allowing one to peer down a looking glass and witness the life forms responsible for disease. It amazes me that 140 years later, we are still diagnosing both the presence and the type of infection by methods largely unchanged from those he developed. Before we knew what infection Christopher had, we took samples of blood, sputum and urine. We then coloured these bodily fluids using the crystal violet dye in the Gram stain and looked at the results using powerful microscopes. This process is still difficult, inaccurate and time-consuming. Many patients with severe infection will not have the bugs identified until they are either recovered or dead. There are a number of new approaches that can improve upon this process. One method identifies tiny fragments of genetic material (DNA or RNA) and then searches a complex electronic library to identify whether these sequences are from a known bug. Another explodes apart tiny fragments of microbes from samples, shoots laser lights at them and analyses their relative weights and reflections to identify fragments that correspond with known microbes.

All of these tests, no matter how accurate, look only at what is there. They do not identify what is significant and what is causing disease. This is important because many microbes are commensals, bacteria that not only live with us peacefully on a day-to-day basis, but actually contribute positively to aspects of our health. Along with a talented team at Cardiff University, I researched the power of the human immune system that, for 6 million years, has responded differently according to the type of infection attacking it. We examined over 300 different immune chemicals that respond when people are infected with different bugs. We then used techniques developed in fields such as economics and artificial intelligence to predict what microbes the human body as a whole was responding to.

Using this new approach of exploiting advanced information analysis from economic systems and the human immune system, ten years after I met Christopher we now have a new method of diagnostic testing for infections. If I could go back in time, I might be able to answer one of Christopher's parents' questions: 'What was causing his disease?' I might be able to tell his mum not only what microbes were there, but what microbes were causing him to die, and help make sense of his story.

~

Five-year-old Sam bounded into the hospital wearing a bright green T-shirt with a dinosaur on the front. Her mum explained how Sam was obsessed with dinosaurs, so much so that they regularly took her to a restaurant that provided crayons and a prehistoric drawing to colour in. Since eating at the restaurant the day before, Sam had developed diarrhoea. When her mum noticed it contained bright streaks of red blood, she brought her to hospital. This was the right thing to do: twelve hours later Sam had severe kidney failure, requiring her to have dialysis.

It is quite likely that Sam had developed an infection from the chicken she had eaten. The type of infection was one that did not take up the purple Gram stain dye, so we knew it wasn't a Gram-positive infection. The other, Gram-negative bacteria have a cell wall that initiates a complex waterfall of immune reactions that gets increasingly magnified as it continues. The type of Gram-negative bug with which Sam was infected was called *Escherichia coli 0157* (a particularly nasty subtype of *E. coli*). This vicious microbe is sometimes found in poultry products and it triggers a dramatic process of physiological and chemical activation, expansion and amplification that, if untempered, can result in kidney failure, heart failure, leaking lungs, bleeding from all surfaces and, ultimately, death at a frightening speed. This is the start of the snowball run and how Sam went from a smiling dinosaur-loving girl to a critically ill patient in just a few hours. The variable that prevents this process occurring with each and every bug we encounter is the host response – the person.

The body's immune system has a number of feedback loops that, like a thermostat in a house, normally allow the 'temperature' of an immune reaction to be just right for killing and inhibiting bacteria and preventing them from continuing their fight against the body. This isn't always the case. If the thermostat's temperature is set too 'cool', then the microbes can grow rapidly and the infection worsens. This may happen, for example, when people are taking powerful drugs, such as steroids, that dampen down the immune system to control diseases such as rheumatoid arthritis. Similarly, if too 'hot', then multi-organ failure can occur, not directly due to the bug but due instead to the very immune reactions that your body is developing. In Sam's case, her immune system got too hot because of the extra-strong signals that the *Escherichia coli 0157* can send out. While we still do not fully understand why this occurs, we do know that some people are pre-programmed to be too 'hot' and some too 'cold'.

Even before the landmark Human Genome Project had mapped all of the genes in the human genome by 2001, it was clear that even minor differences in the genetic blueprint present inside each of us can radically change not only the risks but also the outcomes of disease. This is starkly clear in conditions such as cystic fibrosis. Here, a single spelling error in the genetic code results in a severe life-limiting disease. This one spelling mistake leads to an average life expectancy for someone with cystic fibrosis of just forty years. Thanks to developments in treatment and organ transplantation, the last patient I cared for with this devastating disease – a fiercely strong, inspiring and independent 45-year-old lady – underwent a successful lung transplant and went on to live a healthy life.

This dramatic genetic roll of the dice is very much the exception rather than the rule. More commonly, genetic variation leads to differential levels of risks and outcomes described in terms of probabilities rather than certainties. For example, having the genetic variation BRCA1 leads to a doubling of the risk of developing breast cancer in a woman's lifetime, but around 50 per cent of women with the BRCA1 gene do not develop breast cancer.

The ways in which genetic make-up influences infection are slowly becoming clear. Firstly, there are distinct variations associated with an increased risk of developing certain infectious diseases. The most well described is the reduction in risk of contracting malaria in patients who have the relatively harmless sickle cell trait. Rather than having the full disease of sickle cell, which causes serious health issues, 25 per cent of people from West Africa have the sickle cell trait, which entails only half of the genetic faults of the full disease. This causes few symptoms but it radically reduces the chances of the protozoan *Plasmodium* entering human red blood cells and causing malaria. This is a clear example of how a 'disease' in the strictest sense can be an adaptive or helpful change when viewed through the prism of human evolution. The disadvantages of sickle cell trait are outweighed by the benefits of reduced infection rates of malaria.

These adaptions are context-specific. Therefore, the relative advantages of sickle cell trait in low-prevalence malaria areas, such as Western Europe, disappear and instead people are left with the minor disadvantages of sickle cell trait. The most striking example of this context shifting is in the hugely increased incidence of diabetes in populations originating from the Indian subcontinent. In human evolutionary history, the ability to maintain high blood sugars in the face of poor food availability was a selective advantage. It was achieved through developing resistance to the hormone responsible for controlling blood sugar, insulin. Insulin resistance is today a major component in the development of type 2 diabetes, five times more common in the Indian ethnographic population compared with the global average and leading to a huge burden of death and suffering. Genetics similarly influence the chances of developing common bacteria diseases like the pneumonia that infected Christopher.

The variation in risks of developing infectious disease is important, but the variation in response to disease is even more noteworthy. People respond radically differently to the presence of foreign microbes. In a brave series of experiments in 2014, American researchers injected the major component of Gram-negative bacteria cell walls, lipopolysaccharides, into healthy volunteers under close medical supervision. Most of these volunteers had few ill effects, developing only a mild temperature. Some of the volunteers felt rather unwell, analogous to having a nasty cold. However, a small number of the volunteers developed signs suggestive of early sepsis. Sam's dramatic illness after food poisoning may have been a graphic illustration of this variation: although the bug itself was one causing a strong immune signal, it may have been the combination with Sam's genetic propensity that led to her critical illness.

If the continued presence of microbes were left unchecked, the volunteers who became unwell are likely to be the people who would start dying from their own body's response to infection. This study is important because it informs us how to direct treatment towards the people at the highest risk. It is also of great importance in terms of clinical research, allowing emerging treatments to be tested on people most likely to benefit. Sadly, this has come too late for some promising new drug treatments. Many have fallen by the wayside, useless without personalised medicine to help target their use to populations most likely to benefit. For most patients, including Christopher and Sam, we are left with just one group of drugs that could save them: antibiotics.

~

In 1928, the scientist Alexander Fleming returned from a family holiday in his native Scotland to his lab in St Mary's Hospital, London. He had left in a hurry a few weeks earlier and so, on opening the thick wooden laboratory door, was confronted by a rather untidy room strewn with a number of plates on which he had been growing bacteria for his research. This would turn out to be the most useful mess in history. After examining colonies of a common skin bacteria, *Staphylococcus aureus*, he noted that an environmental mould called *Penicillium notatum* had contaminated the samples. Rather than ruining his series of experiments, this lapse in rigour would change the world of medicine for ever. Around the mould, like a perimeter wall, were areas of clarity where *Staphylococcus aureus* was not able to grow. The realisation of the mould's ability to prevent growth of bacteria led to the birth of the world's first known antibiotic, soon to be known as penicillin. This serendipitous mistake would save the lives of around 200 million people globally in the ninety years that followed.

Medical science rarely operates at an effective pace and it would be fourteen years until, in 1942, Anne Miller, a 33-year-old nurse from New York, became the first patient to be treated with this new drug. She was in a New Haven hospital, critically ill due to an infection caused by the same streptococcal bacteria that infected Christopher. She developed the infection following a miscarriage, but thanks to 5.5 g of penicillin delivered by Merck, a pharmaceutical company helping to mass-produce the experimental drug, Anne would survive. Within twenty-four hours of first receiving penicillin, her condition rapidly improved, her infection relented and she went on to become a proud mother of three boys. She died in 1999 at the age of ninety. The delay in the clinical use of penicillin was largely due to the complexity of transitioning from small-scale research production of the drug to a supply chain capable of reliably being used in healthcare. This metamorphosis required the skills of the triad of Fleming, Howard Florey (a professor of pathology at Oxford University) and his colleague Ernst Boris Chain (a German-born biochemist) to translate Fleming's mistake into a tangible treatment to benefit humanity.

Some ninety years after Fleming's breakthrough, this class of drugs is still at the forefront of therapies used every day to fight bacterial infections. We now have around fifteen classes of antibiotics that attack microbes in one of five main ways. Many destroy the tough outer cell wall of microbes; others stop its production altogether. Some hijack the DNA-production machinery inside each cell or interfere with the final steps in protein production. Some antibiotics destroy the complex membrane structure inside microbes that co-ordinate and carry out essential processes.

Like most street fights, there are strong defences against these attacks. Bacteria have found ingenious methods of deactivating, destroying or avoiding the substances used in antibiotics. As bacteria produce offspring every four minutes, random genetic mutations rapidly accumulate. Some of these accidents result in the ability to neutralise antibiotics. We call this the development of resistance. Unsurprisingly, these bacteria are more likely to survive and so pass on these resistance genes to the next generation. They can even be physically passed – through the movement of protein packages called plasmids – to other bacteria that lack these abilities.

The development of resistance can be an issue within individual patients. People can improve initially after receiving antibiotics only to deteriorate further when those same antibiotics become no longer effective after the microbes become resistant. These resistant strains are a bigger issue in certain populations or geographical areas. Although antibiotic resistance is nothing new, it is compounded by the limited number of new antibiotic classes discovered over the last thirty years. In fact, there has been just one: teixobactin. Although hailed as a breakthrough, this drug still simply acts on a microbe's cell wall. This is similar to some existing antibiotic classes, although teixobactin does so using a different mechanism, blocking the production of cellular fats.

Pharmaceutical development is being outpaced by microbial antibiotic resistance. Big Pharma is losing against the little bugs. There are strains of both tuberculosis and the most common bacteria causing bloodstream infections, *Escherichia coli* (what infected Sam), that are resistant to all known antibiotics. Antibiotic resistance has been highlighted by the World Health Organization as the most pressing threat to global safety, and international initiatives aim to support the development of new antimicrobial classes. This work is slow, expensive and prone to raising false hope. In addition, the need to treat severe infections for only a short, finite period poses difficult financial challenges to pharmaceutical companies, which need to recuperate the high costs of drug development. Either you get better and so need no further drugs with the associated costs, or you do not and you die. While these returns can be easily modelled when developing a drug to treat a common lifelong disease such as rheumatoid arthritis, an effective treatment that cures a patient of an uncommon bacterial infection is not fiscally attractive. The world would not relish a return to the pre-antibiotic era, where severe infection has no effective treatment other than time, hope or death of the patient. Therefore, global co-operation is needed, and central governmental funding for research into new antibiotics is essential along with engagement with industry.

Antibiotics are one of the most common drugs used in the ICU in our fight for the critically ill. While the concept of antimicrobial resistance is important to appreciate, when treating a critically ill patient with multi-organ failure from severe infection, there is little choice other than to reach for the strongest, broadest-spectrum antibiotic that will effectively kill a wide range of bacteria. The medical literature supports the early use of these powerful antibiotics, finding that a delay of just one hour in administration is associated with an increase in the likelihood of death by nearly 8 per cent. When the chances of death in severe infection are already 20 per cent, no one wants this additional risk.

These studies are not perfect, and there are some who

question whether the use of such strong antibiotics that effectively smash bacteria to bits may be harmful in people who are already so unwell. We know that it is often a patient's own body's reaction to infection that leads to organ failure and death rather than the pathogen itself. Therefore it follows that agents that increase this immune activation through release of microbiological fragments may cause harm. Despite these theoretical concerns, international guidelines rightly promote the early administration of antibiotics to those with severe infection, alongside early 'source control' where the infectious focus should be removed as quickly as possible.

~

Just five days after walking through our doors critically unwell, Sam was a very different little girl. The powerful antibiotics she had been given into her veins were the right ones to fight her infection. Her body had reacted in a violent fashion to the *E. coli* but this time it had paid off. The drugs we had been using to help Sam's heart squeeze were first reduced before we were able to stop them altogether. The whirling kidney machine next to Sam's bed that had kept her awake for days fell silent. Her mum had never imagined she would be so grateful to see fresh urine, but as it collected in Sam's catheter bag, she knew her daughter's kidneys had been resurrected. Intensive care had given Sam the right diagnosis and the right drugs at the right time. It had given her time for her body to recover. It had given this little girl another shot at becoming a big girl. Sam waved goodbye to us wearing that same dinosaur T-shirt that had caught my eye five days earlier. We would never see Sam again, and that was a very good thing.

Christopher's story, unfortunately, had a different outcome. Three weeks after becoming unwell, he was transported by plane back to his home in the United Kingdom, still unconscious and on a life-support machine. By this time, the amount of oxygen able to pass through his lungs was so low that he needed to be put onto a machine that would breathe for him over 300 times per minute. This machine used a method of delivering oxygen more like what happens when a dog pants than what normal human breathing can achieve. Although the original antibiotics given were ones known to effectively kill the bacteria that had crept into his lungs in Africa, Christopher was dying. He was dying not from the direct action of the *Streptococcus pneumoniae*, an ancient bacteria older than human history. He was dying from his body's reaction to that bacteria weeks after the initial infection. His body was killing him, and very sadly there was little we could do to intervene.

I remember the day Christopher had his eighteenth birthday while in intensive care. As the candles danced and the balloons floated, surrounded by photos of the good times in his life, Christopher became thinner and weaker. He had regained consciousness a few weeks earlier after his sedation had been reduced. Now, during the ever-shorter lucid periods, he would turn and ask his mum: 'What more can

I do?' Twelve weeks after coughing in the shadows of the roof of Africa, Christopher died while his family took it in turns to hold his hand. He had died of sepsis. Even using the best treatments we have, one in five patients with this severe form of sepsis will not survive.

Ten years later I would visit Christopher's family at home. The red wool is still tied to the roof of his dad's car. We will explore the impact that death through critical illness can have on families later in this book. For now, it is sufficient to say that I will never forget Christopher's case, and in the months and years that followed he would often come into my thoughts when I met patients with severe infection. This would give me a heightened sense of urgency to treat infection early and aggressively.

~

On my first day back at work after a family holiday in France, I met Catrin, a 25-year-old patient who was in a very difficult place. Her family described how their daughter was perfectly healthy apart from occasional episodes of eczema and cold sores. A week earlier, she had developed a temperature, her breathing had become difficult and she started coughing up phlegm. By the time I met her on a cloudy Monday morning, Catrin was suffering with lung and kidney failure and was on a life-support machine. Her family had been told that she might not survive. Despite already having been administered the strongest antibiotics, her lungs were getting worse rather than better. Something did not feel right about this. Why was Catrin not improving with treatment as Sam had done?

Occam's razor is a principle much loved in medicine, first described by the Franciscan friar William of Ockham. It states that the simplest answer to a problem is most often the correct one. Why was Catrin not getting better following treatment for her infection? The simple answer would be that Catrin did not have an infection. But, if so, why was her body behaving as if she did?

Many conditions cause symptoms that suggest infection but are not due to infection. If you were to have a severe car accident, in the twenty-four hours that followed you would develop a rapid heart rate, your temperature would go up, and the blood markers that are used to diagnose infection would become elevated. This 'acute phase response' mimics severe infection. The key to distinguishing whether the symptoms are the result of an infection or not is knowledge of the patient's story. In Catrin's case, we explored her story in detail with her family, interrogated her tests and examined every inch of her body.

When people visit an ICU, they often comment on its complexity. Filled with beeping machines, multiple drug infusions and specialist monitors, it can be a daunting place. The reality is somewhat different. While the technology is important, as we have learnt, the most important element that intensive care offers is far simpler: time. Time to dedicate the efforts of a whole team to a small number of people most in need. Time to explore their story, time to interrogate every one of their dozens of tests, and time to examine their body in immaculate detail both inside and out. We also give patients time, through the use of machines, to allow their body to get better by itself. Voltaire once said, 'The art of medicine consists in amusing the patient while nature cures the disease.' This is often true, even in the complex environment of the ICU.

Catrin's family told us that she would commonly be troubled by cold sores, often in bouts and for long periods of time. She would be quite tired when they occurred, but strangely no one else in the family would develop them. In addition, we noticed that the sputum she was producing was bloodstained, as was her urine. Although her infection blood markers were high, they were not as high as we would expect in such a severe infection. Despite repeated attempts to isolate bugs from her blood, urine and sputum, nothing was found. We began to think that this was a condition masquerading as infection – a traitor in the ranks.

The immune processes in many different conditions are very similar. Rather than direct the immune anger towards an external pathogen, the body can occasionally develop autoimmunity and direct attacks against normal healthy tissues. There are different types of these auto-immune diseases, often occurring in clusters in the same patient. Eczema, hay fever, asthma, diabetes and vitiligo are common autoimmune conditions found in millions of people. There is also a spectrum of severe autoimmune diseases, including a subset called vasculitis, where the targets of the immune system's misplaced zest are the very blood vessels that carry immune cells. As blood vessels are found throughout the body, this condition can mimic different diseases, from strokes to heart attacks. It can also mimic an infection causing lung and kidney failure, the very problem that Catrin had.

Every day that Catrin spent in intensive care the family at her bedside would encounter a sea of new faces. Although the nursing staff soon became familiar, they struggled to remember the names of the physiotherapists, dieticians, pharmacists, occupational therapists and speech therapists, to name but a few. By her third day, more people had cared for Catrin than were in her entire extended family. A key aspect of intensive care medicine is the role of the intensive care doctor as the conductor of a complex and ever-changing orchestra of healthcare, since it is the hard work and dedication of these other professionals, not only the doctors, that results in patient survival.

Visiting specialist teams also play an important part in looking after critically ill patients. These are experts in their fields of interest, be it cardiology or neurology, whom we ask for advice to produce a single co-ordinated care plan. In Catrin's case, we asked for help from Dr Nash, a rheumatologist with vast experience in treating autoimmune diseases. Renowned for their clinical acumen (plus their pleasant bedside manner and inquiring nature), rheumatologists specialise in diseases that touch almost every element of the body. Dr Nash was the ICU's go-to man for these weird and mysterious diseases that require a combined effort to both diagnose and treat effectively. After visiting Catrin, Dr Nash, dressed in his trademark tweed jacket and black spectacles, meticulously went over the patient's story once again and reviewed the results of the tests that we had ordered. With a glint in his eye, he agreed with our suspicion. This was not an infection, but a disease where the immune system was attacking itself. The combination of mouth ulcers, haemoptysis (coughing up blood) and kidney failure pointed towards a disease called Behçet's syndrome, which causes inflammation of the blood vessels. Our machines had given us the time to dedicate to Catrin, and we could now make sense of her story.

Why would the human immune system attack itself, though? This is a key question asked by researchers over the past hundred years. The German immunologist and Nobel laureate, Paul Ehrlich, coined the term 'horror autotoxicus', or the horror of self-toxicity, to describe the body's aversion to immunological self-destruction. Although we do not yet have a clear answer, we have hints at what may influence this process. Most notably, the immunologist David Strachan published his 'clean hypothesis' in 1989, and this has since formed a guiding principle in applied research. It outlines that, in 6 million years of human evolution, the development of the immune system is one of the greatest achievements. It is so important to our survival as a species that it has allowed us to exist alongside other life. We not only live side by side with millions of other life forms, but embrace an ecosystem of microscopic life living on and under our skin. For the vast majority of this time, it was essential to combat the daily barrage of infections from parasites, worms, bacteria and viruses. Following the first agricultural revolution 10,000 years ago, life changed for *Homo sapiens*. No longer nomadic, we lived in settled, cleaner communities. We ate more grain and fewer infected animal parts. This 'progress' has continued to the point where today our homes are relative sanctuaries of sterility in which we interact with animals far less, and wash our hands, our clothes and each other multiple times per day with microbe-killing substances.

Nowadays our immune system is bored. And instead of directing its anger towards external threats, this lack of training through childbirth into adulthood results in an immune system that can turn on itself. Occasionally, this produces no more than dry skin and an itchy nose; in some cases, it would result in death were it not for intensive care medicine.

Sometimes even medicine is not enough. Despite having access to the antibiotic treatments discovered by Fleming and the full support of the ICU, Christopher had sadly died. I wish there were an easy explanation why. It was a deadly combination of a powerful bug and Christopher's immune system not being suited to defeating it in a fight even with the best treatments we could offer. In contrast, Sam's dramatic decline and recovery can be traced back to what we have learnt about different subtypes of infection and the human blueprint that underlies our individual immune responses to these organisms. Sam was fortunate in that her immune response was just right and – thanks to early, effective diagnosis and treatment – she survived.

In Catrin's case, the key piece of the puzzle was the diagnosis and the ability to look beyond infection as a cause of her problems. A correct diagnosis not only allows for the correct treatment to be delivered but also for the incorrect treatments to be withdrawn. After discussion with the rheumatologists, we were confident enough to stop Catrin's antibiotics and to start powerful drugs that would halt her immune system in its tracks – an avalanche shield to stop the snowball of her immune system from running away any further. Twenty-four hours after using the steroid drug methylprednisolone, Catrin was given a designer drug called rituximab. A drug like this is produced artificially by scientists after painstaking analysis and protein modelling. Designer drugs are made to be just the right shape and size to fit into tiny gaps, or receptors, on the surface of cells to either activate or block their function. In Catrin's case, the drug prevented her immune cells from producing the antibodies causing her disease. She started to improve. Her lungs needed less oxygen, her kidneys started producing urine and the cold sores on her lips regressed. We were using modern pharmaceutical technology, combined with 6-million-year-old acumen, to blow on the porridge of her immune system. Within seven days Catrin was back home with her family. And that is why I love this job.

3

Skin and Bones

Damage to the scaffolding of life

One attraction of medicine as a career is the global passport it offers to doctors, allowing them to apply their skills anywhere in the world. I was fortunate to travel to the beautiful city of Perth, Western Australia, with my young family to spend one year working at one of the busiest trauma hospitals in the world. The adventure started with a 24-hour plane journey during which I desperately tried to entertain my energetic, wriggling eighteen-month-old daughter. The reward was to spend time in a sun-kissed city perched on the peppermint-blue Swan river. It was a great year.

Twelve months after the wheels of the plane met the hot Australian tarmac, we returned home. I often ask myself why – in the face of better pay, shorter hours, interesting medicine, beautiful scenery and perfect weather – we returned. The answer is clear: we returned home for the same reason that Rob's dad – whom I would meet during the time I spent in Perth – spent an hour sitting in silence in his car outside the Royal Perth Hospital. We returned home to be close to our family. Rob's dad desperately wanted to do the same. But he did not. He could not. Not yet.

~

An hour earlier, the noise must have been deafening as the explosion ripped through the wooden house in a quiet suburb just south of the peaceful Swan river. As the pressure wave reverberated, the roof was torn off like the top of an old blister. The costs of the damage would exceed £200,000. A toddler was seen running across the debris-strewn, scorched lawn. Behind him was his four-year-old sister. The five adults in the house were all injured but none as badly as Rob. As the rescue sirens of the Australian emergency services sounded, Rob lay unconscious, breathing heavily and with severe burns across his face, arms and back. The street name of the drug that Rob had been trying to make in his improvised laboratory was exactly what his injuries needed: ice. It was one of the biggest meth-lab drug explosions ever recorded.

We thankfully see very few injuries following explosions in civilian health services. Training with the American military during my short time in the Royal Air Force opened my eyes to what could happen. Blast injuries are broadly divided into three stages. Primary injuries result from the blast wave produced by high-energy explosions. This force propagates through space, affecting air- and fluid-filled body regions. Injuries that can result include ruptured bowels, lungs, eyes and eardrums. Death can quite easily occur from this invisible yet deadly force alone. Secondary injuries are caused by flying projectiles carried by the pressure wave. As force = mass × speed, even innocent objects can be transformed into deadly weapons. A chair, a table, a mobile phone or even another person's severed limb would cause significant injury should they impact against your head at 300 mph. Finally, tertiary injuries happen when your body is thrown forcibly into static objects in the vicinity.

~

I am very accustomed to the yearly ebb and flow of patients through my intensive care unit. As the autumn trees start to sweat white frost, I meet patients with influenza. Six months later, I will care for patients rescued from drowning in the warmer summer months. These stories are cyclical but, for the families involved, these are all individual, unpredictable, tragic events – 'black swan events'. This term describes outlier occurrences, such as the terrorist attacks of 9/11 or even Brexit on a global scale. The etymology behind the term 'black swan events' stems from the sixteenth-century belief that all swans were white until the expedition of Willem de Vlamingh in 1697 to the Swan river area in Western Australia – where Rob now lives. While exploring the area, de Vlamingh described a large water bird with black plumage and a bright red bill. It would later be called *Cygnus atratus*, or the black swan. In 2007, the term was borrowed by the Lebanese-American author Nassim Nicholas Taleb who uses it in his book, *The Black Swan*, to describe unpredictable events that have wide-ranging, society-changing effects. He argued that, while humans are poor at specific future predictions, unlikely events will occur and dramatically alter our lives. Overall the likelihood of any one specific black swan event is extremely low, but just like predicting intensive care admissions, the overall likelihood of one occurring at some time is very high.

One such event happened on 12 October 2002. In Kuta, on the Indonesian island of Bali, a terrorist explosion killed 202 people, injuring a further 209. Within hours of the tragedy, survivors with severe burns were arriving at the Royal Perth Hospital as the nearest support facility. In total, the hospital cared for twenty-eight patients, many benefiting from the breakthrough 'spray-on skin' developed by the pioneering surgeon, Fiona Wood. This black swan event paved the way for the hospital to become a leading burns centre, a place that would give Rob the best chance of survival.

As Rob arrived in the emergency department, the smell of burnt flesh lingered at the back of my throat like a beach barbecue. Seeing the severe facial burns, our first concern was the imminent swelling that occurs in the minutes and hours after a heat injury. There are a number of markers that signify a patient's airway may have been damaged from superheated gas. A change in the quality of their voice, black, sooty sputum or singed nasal hairs are all worrying signs. Unless a patient's airway is secured early, rapid and severe swelling may make breathing impossible just minutes later. If left too long, the only way to access a patient's airway to prevent them from suffocating to death would be through the front of their neck. Every intensive care doctor's worst nightmare is doing emergency surgery in this scenario at the bedside with just a scalpel and a plastic tube. You have 120 seconds to perform a delicate operation that normally takes an hour, with no prior warning, no preparation, only the most basic of equipment and an outcome that will be either life or death.

Thankfully, this wasn't needed on this occasion. After receiving anaesthetic and paralysis drugs, Rob's airway was secured through his mouth just in time. I looked at his vocal cords using the curved metal blade of a laryngoscope, designed to push the soft tissues of the mouth out of the way while illuminating the path to the vocal cords using a light at its tip. This revealed red and swollen tissues with flecks of black carbonised soot coating the lining of his airway. Despite Rob being placed onto a life-support machine, the amount of oxygen in his blood stayed dangerously low.

Toxic fumes, including carbon monoxide, can cause low oxygen levels after a patient is rescued from a fire in a confined space. However, we were suspicious that the strong blast wave had caused direct damage to Rob's lungs. An urgent chest X-ray confirmed our concerns. His lungs appeared bright white as his delicate air sacs had become filled with fluid following the blast injury. More worrying was the thick rim of air between the inside of Rob's chest wall and his lung surface. Called a pneumothorax, this had occurred when the roof had been torn from the house as the explosion caused a rapid expansion of gas. The same expansion had occurred inside Rob's lungs. This rapid pressure increase ruptured the walls of the air sacs, causing a leak of air into the pleural space. The tissue around this blast hole had formed a makeshift one-way valve. With every breath we pushed into Rob, more air would flow into this space. Unless this was relieved, the pressure would get ever higher, eventually causing Rob's heart to stop beating.

I took a scalpel and made a cut deep into Rob's skin down to the gristle surface of a rib at the bottom of his armpit. Using my finger, I felt around for the familiar, narrow space between his ribs, breaking down the muscle fibres as I pushed from side to side. As my finger popped through the final tough layer on the inside of his ribcage, a gush of blood-filled air signalled I had found the correct space. Sweeping my finger in a circle around the inside surface of the ribs, I felt Rob's soft lung expanding and contracting with every breath and the beat of his heart nudging the tip of my finger.

Once Rob's initial life-threatening injuries had been stabilised, the extent of his burns could be assessed. After a careful examination, we calculated 20 per cent burns of his body, mostly of partial thickness but also some full-thickness burns involving all three layers of the skin. It was clear that Rob would need surgical treatment and skin grafting.

Skin is our biggest and most important immune structure. Stretched out flat, it covers an area the size of two large dining-room tables. It teems with life, harbouring more than a thousand different types of bacteria and fungi, the exact combination being as unique to you as your fingerprint. Wipe this habitat clean with disinfectant and just twelve hours later your exact microbial fingerprint will respawn as if using a time machine.

Your skin is the first barrier that foreign intruders encounter and the toughest for them to overcome. The development of significant infection caused by multi-drug-resistant organisms is almost universal following major burns. Not only does skin stop things getting in, but it provides essential scaffolding to the body, keeping the parts of you inside of you. Within minutes of a serious burn, huge shifts occur in the fluid compartments of your body. As much as 200 ml of fluid per hour is lost after nature's finest waterproof coat no longer functions. As well as losing fluid, patients with burns radiate huge amounts of heat. The high ambient temperature maintained in specialist burns units to compensate for this hits unsuspecting visitors as though they had stepped off an airplane having landed in Australia's Red Centre.

Although we replace lost fluids using a careful mathematical formula, much leaks out from cell connections struggling from the effects of such significant trauma. This leads to swelling throughout the body and even within the organs. Combined with a dramatic increase in metabolism (the chemical reactions happening in the body), organ failure in patients with severe burns is common. Massive muscle and tissue breakdown compounds this by producing high levels of the muscle protein myoglobin. After being transported to the kidneys, these large molecules lodge in the small pores of the renal system, leading to kidney failure.

As Rob lay motionless in the ICU, his dad was fighting a battle of his own. When he heard the news about his son, he did what any parent would do and drove quickly to the hospital. He parked his car just metres away from the ICU on that hot, humid evening during one of the hottest years on record. As the key turned, silencing the car's engine, he hesitated. A thousand possible scenarios flooded his mind. After twenty minutes of indecision came harsh clarity. He turned the key again and the car's engine added to the heat of the summer night. Rob's dad drove home and wouldn't see his son for another five days. Years later he told a national newspaper of his dilemma that night: 'You either go in there and be a father or you stay outside and be a police commissioner. You can't be both.'

Years after meeting Rob, I reconnected with father and son. Although Rob had needed multiple skin grafts following the explosion, his lung injury quickly improved, and within a week he was discharged from the ICU. Days later, his father hugged his son for the first time since the accident.

They both realised during that embrace that the journey ahead would be long and hard. They were right. A poignant image of a grief-stricken yet strong police commissioner visiting his criminal son was soon all over the front pages of newspapers across Australia.

~

Think about the worst mistake you have ever made. It may be something that only you know. It could be illegal, immoral or just unfair. It may have happened yesterday or fifty years ago. No matter how awful this mistake may be, it is not the sum total of you. You are not your worst mistake. Most of us, through good fortune, will get away with having made mistakes in our lives. The text you sent on your phone while driving last week did not lead to a disaster. For someone, somewhere, it did. For that person, they will be seen through the prism of that mistake for evermore. They are no different from you apart from happenstance.

I have treated a lot of people who have made mistakes. I have cared for paedophiles, drug dealers, murderers, rapists and wife-beaters. I've cared for people who have smoked and drunk themselves to death. Is this right? Should we still use limited resources, time and money on those who have made life a misery for others? Yes. Yes, we should.

For a start, the 'facts' that we are presented with in intensive care are often wrong. When I was working in Australia, I remember treating an Aboriginal lady who had previously had a heart transplant. She was also an alcoholic. She was admitted after a car accident caused, I was told, by her drink-driving. This had resulted in the deaths of her three grandchildren travelling in the back of her car. I remember feeling angry at the resources that she had benefited from through her transplant compared with the waste of innocent lives from her selfish actions. After she died from her severe injuries, I felt cheated by the fact that she would not face justice.

Weeks later while completing paperwork related to her death, I was told that her blood-alcohol level on admission had actually been zero. Speaking with the family, they described how she had not been able to afford the medications needed to prevent rejection of her transplanted heart while single-handedly caring for her three grandchildren. She had actually died of a heart attack at the wheel due to her inability to afford the anti-rejection tablets. It was not drink-driving. We couldn't offer a cure or a heroic save for that lady, but we could offer reality and truth. The family were grateful that we had 'made sense of her story'.

Even if troublesome facts about a patient's past are true, care is not a commodity that should be sanctioned through worth. Using withdrawal of care as a punishment is a slippery slope to a society that loses respect for human life. Care is not a weapon to wield against people's choices, no matter how foolish they are. While healthcare rationing should consider factors affecting the likelihood of success, this should not be based around assigning value to choices.

If society chose not to treat heavy smokers or alcoholics, should it still care for the obese, the inactive, motorbike riders, adventure-sports junkies or those who do not tie their shoelaces correctly? Responsibility is a two-way street but society owes a duty of care to all, including those who make bad choices.

The more I speak with people who have made poor 'choices' in life, the more sceptical I become about the role that free will plays in their demise. Although I get applauded and congratulated for achievements in life, can they really be traced back to choices made only by me? I did not choose to be born into a loving family, with enough money to buy books, in a country with free education, in a century where infant mortality rates allowed me to live. I didn't choose the balance of neurotransmitters in my brain that enables me to understand science yet not fall prey to drug addiction or violence. Even if I were able to make the 'right choices', these are a grain of sand buried below a desert of opportunity that I was given. This viewpoint is supported by neurocognitive evidence underpinning Sam Harris' description of 'the illusion of free will'. Functional MRI studies, scanning areas of the brain involved in cognition, now show that subconscious processes predetermine our choices long before we are even aware of 'us' making a decision. This is simply more evidence that care should not be given according to worth. It also makes me consider what led me to choose medicine as a career.

My path to becoming an intensive care consultant was as tortuous as the naive, teenage wish I made about becoming a doctor. Far from being a long-thought-out life choice, if it hadn't been for my careers tutor life may have been very different. Looking up from my record, she said: 'So you have written here that you want to be Fox Mulder from *The X-Files* television programme. Is that a joke?' It wasn't. David Duchovny's character blended science, logic and passion as well as that element of mystery to keep viewers coming back. I did not realise at that time, but treating your mum, your child or your grandmother in critical care today fulfils virtually all of these old dreams that I had as a teenage boy. The unknown element in my medical research has made me stay in the hospital not only late at night but year after year. The mysteries in critical illness can be big, such as why some patients will die quickly yet others will live despite having the same disease. Your own chances of survival depend on a diverse range of factors including your median income, adding to the worries that a widened socio-economic gap has real-world health implications even for those who stay in an intensive care bed. On a day-to-day basis, the mysteries I encounter may be relatively small compared with these challenges, yet they flex my mind more than even the hardest sudoku puzzle.

I still remember as a teenager reading the letter offering me a place at medical school as my hands trembled in both excitement and anticipation. At that moment, I little appreciated just how many examinations lay ahead of me compared with those trailing behind. Twenty years later, the smell of a library book still transports me back to the multitude of undergraduate and major post-graduate examinations, countless essays, dissertations and terrifying clinical tests that I endured to call myself a critical care consultant.

I remember as clearly as a Polaroid photograph the first time I examined a real patient in front of a real doctor. I felt clumsy in my skin as I dropped my stethoscope to the ground before putting it into my ears the wrong way round. As technology has moved on in critical care, I now hardly ever use a stethoscope. But during the recent check-up for our newest family member – a fox-red male cockapoo puppy called Chester – the vet offered his stethoscope to us all to listen to the puppy's heartbeat. After my children had confidently heard the *lub-dub* of Chester's heart valves snapping closed, I again placed the ear pieces in the wrong way round, much to the hilarity of my family, and I was abruptly reminded of the cold sweat I had felt on that grey morning as a nineteen-year-old medical student.

Difficult, costly exams and endless practical assessments have been a regular fixture in the calendar of my life for over twenty years. They come around predictably like seasons – some pleasant and breezy, others cold and harsh. Exams remain an important part of the journey from student to doctor although the old-style, dramatic final exams at the end of medical training have largely gone. Tests of pure recall are still important but they alone cannot be enough to make a good, or even safe, doctor. As medicine stumbles into the age of machine learning and artificial intelligence, it is easy to think that more data and better answers are all that is important. Just as dark shadows are made using the brightest of lights, artificial intelligence brings with it new, difficult questions. Sometimes it is asking the right questions that is first needed before combining multiple simple answers into a complex whole. This is essential for critical care exams where doctors can be bombarded with hundreds of data points simultaneously at the bedside – from blood tests to handwritten notes, X-rays to multiple tracings of the heart. Simply assessing these in isolation is not helpful for critically ill patients; it is the integration of these into a larger whole that is needed.

What sick patients need are doctors who can integrate the complexity of medicine by asking the right questions to start with. With the development of machines such as IBM's supercomputer Watson, even this human integration can be replicated. Knowing that my medical training cost the public over £500,000, should society instead rely on a robot without a heart or a human doctor *with* one? There is much more to my role as an intensive care doctor than simply providing a diagnosis or a treatment plan. If that were all I did then perhaps the robot would be the right choice. My strength as a human doctor lies in my ability to orchestrate a complex, messy, human care team to focus on a unique, human patient. Knowing the answers is only one part of the solution. Long gone *should* be the days of painted portraits showing a single, eminent, white, middle-class man hanging on the walls in hospital corridors. These need to be replaced by teams of diverse people working together with a much better gender balance. This, combined with the humanity to communicate with patients, families and staff, is what makes me (currently) more valuable than Watson.

The endless exams that plagued my medical training focused on questions with a single, certain answer. Yet intensive care frequently deals with uncertainty and so, while harder to design, exams should assess a human doctor's ability to ask and answer questions where there are no clear right or wrong answers. We need to learn to be open to the differences between one's ability to provide an invasive treatment and the more important question of whether it should be provided at all. What I *can* do is not always what I *should* do. Medicine is all about understanding a patient's story. None of the robots I have yet met are very good storytellers, yet the human doctors I work with are.

~

Years after that hot Perth summer, the scene from my window is very different. The first day of March 2018 should have been the start of a new, hopeful spring. Instead it was the slow end of a long, cold winter. It was the day I nearly walked out.

The stresses and strains I experience as a critical care doctor can often be described as having opposed yet parallel tracks. I do not break psychologically due to one big failure or event. Although I remember many patient stories, there are no individuals who haunt or motivate me above all others. Instead, the day I nearly walked out was due to the exact opposite of how successful cycling teams describe their success – thanks to aggregation of marginal gains. I nearly walked out instead due to the aggregation of marginal losses. A lot of little things nearly broke me.

The 'Beast from the East' was a fearsome weather front that caused out-of-season weather chaos across the UK in early March 2018. Instead of purple tulips bursting up through my garden soil readying for spring, the first weekend of March saw sixteen weather-related deaths as the heaviest snowfall in more than thirty-five years was dumped on an ill-prepared UK. This coincided with one of the busiest periods for critical care services ever described, with many ICUs swelling to over 150 per cent of their funded capacities. We had twenty-six beds but forty-six patients. It was an important but tough weekend to be rostered on – especially when, after four days stranded away from home by snow, few staff could get to work let alone leave at the end of a long day. After coping with little food, little sleep and a lot of sick patients, the aggregation of marginal losses erupted inside of me when an urgent phone call warned that a foreign embassy official had just arrived to take one of our sickest patients with a severe skin infection away to a private hospital. I knew that even the journey could result in that patient's death – bumps on the road can cause dangerous changes in blood pressure and lying flat reduces oxygen levels – and yet we were being put under pressure to let the patient go. However, I was too tired to even argue. I should not have even been in work that day. I was only there to help due to the snow. I looked at children building snowmen through the hospital window and wondered what my children were doing. Why not just walk home and not look back? I had given my everything, but that was not enough.

Life has taught me that people who have been hurt are those most likely to hurt others. Yet there is a secret escape route signposted to us by the physician and author Viktor Frankl. After surviving the horrors of the Holocaust he wrote: 'When no longer able to change a situation, we are challenged to change ourselves.' He followed that: 'Between stimulus and response there is a space. In that space is our power to choose our response. In our response lies our growth and our freedom.' Finding the mental space to react with a cool brain instead of a hot head can be hard. But, without it we can easily hurt ourselves and others.

Something kept me from walking out through the door on that snowy day. Perhaps it was free will, perhaps seren-dipity, perhaps a deterministic, mechanistic fate. We spoke to the ill patient's family who had arranged the private-hospital transfer. They were very loving, reasonable, rational and, like me, wanted only what was in their loved one's best interests. They had arranged the transfer not through loss of trust, but through love, the love of a parent for a child who was critically ill while in a country thousands of miles from home. Feeling helpless, the only thing for that parent to have done was to send any support they could. When faced with the reality of the situation, the parents reacted with their cerebral and not adrenal, accepting that their child should stay with us and not travel to London.

After that conversation, I stayed at work and didn't leave for another twelve hours. The aggregation of marginal losses had led me to question my job, my role and my life. But when I remembered the big things, these little things remained small. The big things matter more, and the big things are still winning as I write this today.

How can we improve critical care systems so that I and others like me do not have another day worth quitting over? I have drunk many cups of instant coffee while the latest initiatives have been presented in hospital management meetings. Well-intentioned, fresh-faced graduates arrive, thrust in from the world of hard business, to talk about how business management methods can solve the woes of a hospital in crisis. They pluck strategies developed in the orderly surroundings of Silicon Valley and try to apply them to a tangled emergency department. They use language such as 'lean management' wrenched from the metal fist of

Japan's post-war car industry and try to apply it to a bloodied operating theatre.

It can help medicine when we selectively borrow techniques from safety-conscious industries. Every day my ward round benefits from using crew-resource management theory and checklists founded in aviation. Other strategies can be helpful when trying to improve the efficiency of operating lists, allowing more knee replacement surgeries to be carried out for the same amount of effort. What these industrial standards do not tell us, however, is how critical care should be delivered at 2 a.m. during a surprisingly brutal cold snap. They often cannot deal with the complexity or the variable and human nature of medicine. Your mum may be distraught if her major operation that required a critical care bed were scheduled for 10 p.m. on Boxing Day in order to achieve a target.

These adoptions can leave patients and staff feeling dehumanised. Anyone who has sat on the other side of healthcare as a patient will remember the things that hit home the most: the vending machine that was empty; that uncomfortable seat that you sat on for hours; the way your name was mispronounced. These are very human experiences that touch us through medicine yet cannot be accounted for in a colourful spreadsheet.

I now look towards innovations that focus instead on better experience rather than simply better output. Experience, safety and efficiency can, and should, coexist. When we bring these three things together they complement rather than clash. The strategies needed for running a hospital should be exactly that – ideally designed for running a hospital and not simply borrowed from other industries. Medicine needs to nurture, design and uncover these for itself.

~

The year 2016 was going to be a great one for Gwen and her young family. She loved her job as an art teacher in a local school. It allowed her infectious creativity to be passed on while affording her a lifestyle suitable for watching her three children grow up. By her mid-thirties, Gwen and her husband were ready for their next adventure. The pull of the Welsh coast, combined with their love of coffee, led to plans being drawn on a tablecloth after a bottle of wine one evening. Just one week after I met Gwen, the family were due to open their coffee shop sewn into the coast road around a beautiful rural Welsh village. All that changed with the accident.

The first paramedics to arrive saw a troubling scene. The tangled metal from three separate cars was virtually indistinguishable, like three shades of paint messily mixed together by hand. Gwen's eldest daughter was limping away from the ball of steel, holding onto her grandmother's hand, shaking with shock. 'Where is mummy?' she asked, looking backwards over her shoulder.

Gwen had been a passenger as her mother-in-law drove safely towards a busy junction. What happened next remains unclear but resulted in Gwen being trapped following a major road traffic collision. It took over two hours to get her out safely while the other occupants escaped with only minor injuries. Lying next to her car once she had been freed, covered in foil blankets, Gwen was critically ill. She was unconscious from her trauma and bleeding from a ruptured aorta (the largest blood vessel in the body), and she couldn't breathe due to multiple rib fractures.

Landing in a muddy field next to the small rural hospital where Gwen had been taken, helicopter doctor Dr Owen McIntyre and critical care practitioner Chris Shaw were tasked with transporting her safely to the regional trauma centre. The helicopter team worked as quickly and as smoothly as a Formula 1 pit-stop team yet with far more at stake than an oversized bottle of champagne. Using their specialist training, regular simulation practice and standard operating procedures, they saved Gwen's life. While using his finger and a scalpel, Dr McIntyre drained the blood surrounding Gwen's lungs. Simultaneously, the team prepared equipment to put her onto a life-support machine. Meanwhile, donated blood and clotting products were being squeezed through a strong needle buried deep into Gwen's shoulder bone as her veins were so collapsed due to the cold and her illness. Travelling through her bone marrow vessels, these donated blood products stopped Gwen from bleeding to death. It wouldn't have mattered if Gwen had still been at the roadside, this helicopter team regularly deliver advanced medical interventions while kneeling on tarmac, hammered by the Welsh weather, shaded by tarpaulin, wherever they are needed.

As naked apes, our ability to assess risk is terrible. We tend to overreact to anecdotal stories such as the tale of a surfer attacked by a shark millions of miles away and worry about the same thing happening to us during our holiday swim. We should worry more about the car journey from our home to the airport.

Globally, over 3,000 people die every day from road traffic collisions, that is 1.3 million deaths per year. Of those who survive, 50 million people are left disabled. Road trauma is largely a disease of the young, being the leading cause of death in people aged between fifteen and thirty. Road safety is steadily improving in the Western world. However, the same cannot be said of low- and middle-income countries where – despite having only half of the world's vehicles – more than 90 per cent of all road fatalities occur.

The fact that Gwen had even arrived at hospital alive can be traced back to the English glider industry. George Cayley was an English engineer who created the first seat belt to keep pilots inside gliders during the nineteenth century. Although the first patented seat belt was used to keep tourists safe in New York City taxis in 1885, it was not until the 1950s that Volvo introduced the three-point system used today. This changed the spectrum of injuries we see in critical care today from severe head injuries to mainly thoracic, abdominal and skeletal trauma. The simple act of wearing a seat belt more than halves your chances of dying in a car accident. It works – use it. Every time.

The blood that Gwen had received also had its roots deep in the history books. Many medical advances are derived from the horror of war. The evolution of a blood-transfusion service was one of the most significant medical outcomes of the First World War. Before 1913, only direct person-to-person blood transfusion was routinely used. The millions of soldiers dying from severe bleeding accelerated research into blood storage using chemical additives. It was noted that fruit-derived citrate prevented blood from clotting and later it was discovered that this was due to its ability to bind the calcium needed for coagulation. The capability to maintain liquid blood thus established the first blood bank capable of forward-planning for managing massive blood loss.

As Gwen was loaded into the Airbus EC-145 helicopter, the team noted that she hadn't once moved her legs. Three hours after the accident, far away from the busy roadside, her husband asked me a difficult question while sitting in the relative calm of the ICU. Gwen was in theatre, having a ruptured bowel repaired and a severe spinal injury stabilised. She hadn't moved her legs because her spinal cord had been damaged as a result of multiple fractures of the bones in her spine. Spinal fractures are a major concern when treating patients with serious trauma. Your spinal cord runs half a metre down the middle of your back, from the base of your brain to a level at the top of your hips. This smooth, rope-like structure has a hundred billion nerve cells packed into a space just the width of your little finger. Such is its importance to life that the hard bony case of the spine wraps completely around it, protecting it from damage. In many ways this bony vertebral column can be considered the scaffolding of life. When the spine is itself shattered, shards of bone turn from being a protective structure to a lethal weapon.

This damage had occurred at the level of Gwen's spinal cord responsible for signals being sent to and from her legs. After I had told Gwen's husband what had happened, a brief moment of cotton-white silence hung in the air. His gaze shifted from the floor back to my eyes. He then asked me one of the most difficult questions I had ever been asked: 'What should I tell my children?' I didn't know what to say.

Answering tricky questions is a staple part of my job. 'Will he survive?', 'Should I stay the night?' and 'Will she ever be the same again?' are pleas uttered by loved ones every hour of every day, right now in critical care units all around the world. The answers are universally difficult yet the same regardless of language. I could guess the answers, I could use statistics to quote death rates of 95 per cent in certain situations. However, that would mean little for the patient who defies the odds as that rare one person in twenty who lives. Instead, as critical care doctors, we should answer these impossible questions with honesty: 'I do not know.' These four words are the most underused words in medicine. They hold much power, allowing for hope yet also preparing for grief. They are also hard to say. People want plans, they want certainty, they want answers gained from years of education and experience. And doctors want to give this. Admitting to yourself that uncertainty cannot be eliminated takes guts. 'I don't know' is the most honest, and paradoxically wise, summary that I can offer.

Two years after I met Gwen and her family, I finally had the answer to her husband's question. My family and I had travelled to the ancient capital of Wales, now a market town called Machynlleth. Just a short drive from where Gwen lived, it was a perfect location to get away from busy clinical shifts and to spend time with our family's new puppy. More importantly, it allowed me to visit Gwen's family in their own home.

Were I able to go back in time and answer Gwen's husband's question, it would be much easier. I would say that his children should know that – thanks to the combination of her seat belt, the air ambulance team, blood donors and a host of healthcare workers – Gwen would not only survive her critical illness but she would eventually thrive. That the journey would be long and hard, and her family would play a key part in her recovery. Gwen's husband should tell his children that their mummy was an incredibly brave and strong woman who would not let any stumbles through the fabric of life blunt her fondness for it. He should tell them that, yes, life will change for ever but, although some doors will close, others will open.

It was a pleasure and privilege to be able to see these

things myself when I met Gwen and her family in their home in 2018. Gwen's coffee shop never opened and the accident had indeed changed the family's life dramatically. Despite extensive rehabilitation, Gwen still needs a wheelchair. This is likely to remain the case for the rest of her life but, overall, a busy, happy family life had continued. She told me that she has dark days when she feels just like 'a head on a stick' and that she misses simple things like dancing with her children. Fighting the barriers of disability has also been a huge challenge. Insightfully, she told me how being disabled and exceptional is accepted by the public, yet being disabled and simply 'normal' is more difficult. Paralympians can be celebrities, whereas most disability does not involve being extraordinary but, instead, striving after a new normality.

Gwen echoed Henry Fraser's thoughts from his fantastic book *The Little Big Things*, which describes his life as a young man after a serious spinal injury. Gwen is deeply appreciative of how much others have given of their lives so that she can live her own. But now it is her turn to continue to live her life. Just six weeks after I met her, she opened a new craft shop in her local village, surrounded by the creative outpourings that had helped her through her painful journey. Although the pieces she created in the early days were dark, as the summer approaches, her artwork for sale has now let some light back in.

4

THE HEART

The 2 billion beats of life

As a first-time author, I hope that many people will read and enjoy this book. I hope it gets good reviews. I hope that I can do justice to my patients and my profession. However, one hope rises to the top. It is a hope that I carry with me each day as I travel to work: I hope this book will actually save someone's life. Maybe your dad's or your friend's, your neighbour's or even that of a stranger you are about to meet in the next coffee shop you visit. Let me explain how we can do this together. But first, I'd like you to meet our next patient, The Judge.

Standing six foot tall with a neatly trimmed beard and a deep, considered voice, he was a powerful man in both stature and presence. Following twenty years' practice as a criminal barrister, he had been a circuit judge for nearly eighteen years, trying almost every type of case in the criminal calendar. He had a reputation for a no-nonsense approach, did not suffer fools gladly yet was always fair. Should he be irritable or transiently lose his temper, he always sought to apologise sincerely. When I first met The Judge, he was no longer this larger-than-life character. He had died. In fact, he had died over twenty times in one day.

His story started on a slow Tuesday morning as he was presiding over a criminal compensation hearing. As the defendants listened anxiously, he began to feel unwell. First, he became dizzy as he rose to his feet and his blood failed to reach his brain. Next, he collapsed as the cells in his body were starved of oxygen, before he hit the carpeted courtroom floor with a thud. The court usher, acting swiftly, saw that he was not breathing and nervously placed her small hands on his chest. She pressed down firmly once, and then again and again and again. If you were to listen to the extraordinary audio recording of these eight minutes while The Judge had died, you would hear the usher's caring Welsh tones as she spoke to him while doing cardiopulmonary resuscitation (CPR). It was the first time she had ever called him by his first name.

As the emergency services arrived, The Judge was still receiving effective bystander CPR. The ambulance crew's monitor, attached to his bare skin, sensed the electrical signals produced by his heart and showed a very abnormal pattern often seen during cardiac arrests. The heart's electrical trace should look like the skyline of a typical Welsh valley: a small hill followed by a large mountain, then a valley before one more hill. Instead, the monitor's screen blazed with an erratic pattern, known as ventricular fibrillation (VF), which prevents any co-ordinated, meaningful heart muscle contraction. As a result, no blood could be squeezed out from The Judge's heart. Unless this was fixed quickly, his life would be extinguished for ever.

Although we will soon see how amazing machines and complex drugs offered The Judge a chance to return to his courtroom, these required one precondition: The Judge first needed to arrive in hospital alive. That seems a rather simple concept, but it is a key factor in what is known as the chain of survival. Every year, 30,000 people in the UK will suddenly collapse to the ground having suffered a cardiac arrest. Their hearts will either have stopped beating completely, started fibrillating (jittering) 200 times a minute – as in The Judge's case – or will be unable to pump out any blood despite the electric circuits working correctly. Of every 100 people who suffer a cardiac arrest, around twenty will make it to the hospital alive. Of these twenty, two will eventually return home to a relatively normal life.

Since the inception of intensive care medicine, most controversy has focused on treatments that patients do *not* receive rather than those they do – particularly the withdrawal or withholding of therapies. We make a decision to withdraw life-sustaining treatment, just as when assessing which interventions to use in the first place, based on the patient's best interests. However, whether we should treat patients with CPR is now a formalised process since the introduction of 'do not attempt resuscitation' (DNAR) orders, and these have assumed a special place in the public consciousness even though CPR is often less effective than other optional therapies. By contrast, the decision-making surrounding withholding antibiotics or even emergency surgery – which can have a more significant effect on life or death – is not formalised in the same manner. I am not arguing that additional pieces of paper should be used to delineate every one of the 5,000 potential medical treatments people can receive. Quite the opposite. Communication, shared decision-making and better public understanding cannot be replaced by a photocopied form like the current DNAR orders. Nor should they be, for increased public awareness of what CPR is has not been accompanied by better public understanding of whom it benefits. When used appropriately, CPR prolongs life and cheats death but, all too often, entrenched views and emotional turmoil result in the use of CPR to simply prolong death and cheat on the dignity of life.

Although television medical dramas emphasise chest compressions as the main component of CPR, this is merely one element. As its full name implies, cardiopulmonary resuscitation involves supporting the lungs alongside the heart. When I care for a patient having a cardiac arrest in the emergency department, after confirming the absence of a pulse by pressing my finger on their carotid artery at the side of their neck, I focus on three elements of resuscitation: A, B and C.

'A' relates to a patient's airway, ensuring a free passage from the outside world into their lungs where air becomes breath. We often perform tracheal intubation, inserting a plastic endotracheal tube through the vocal cords into the trachea. Providing a conduit for breath is the most ancient component of CPR, as revealed by stories in the Babylonian Talmud where a lamb with an injury to the neck was rescued by making a hole in the windpipe and inserting a hollow reed. This tradition of using improvised pipe-like structures to bypass obstructions in the trachea continues to this day, with objects as diverse as ballpoint pens and drinking straws having been used to save lives. Advances in airway control continued when the Dutch Humane Society, founded in 1768 to help drowning victims, recommended using bizarre practices including rolling patients upside down in a barrel after water submersion. This was meant to clear the airway of water and any foreign bodies. Unsurprisingly, it was not terribly successful and (hopefully) is no longer used. It took the invention of the laryngoscope by Alfred Kirstein in 1895 before a tube could be reliably inserted into the trachea.

Insertion of endotracheal tubes allows not only block-ages to be bypassed, but importantly enables oxygen-rich air to be forced into a patient's lungs by squeezing an inflatable bag, just as the medical students had used to save Vivi. This 'B' component of CPR provides artificial breathing and hence supplies oxygen to the lungs. The use of inflatable bags attached to oxygen improved upon the recommended technique of inserting a fire-bellows into people's nostrils and anus in the 1500s, hence the term 'blowing smoke up one's arse'. There followed the advent of 'mouth-to-mouth' breathing, with an early description provided by surgeon William Tossach when, on 3 December 1732 at Alloa in Scotland, he resuscitated the coal miner James Blair by using mouth-to-mouth rescue breathing. The worker had been 'in all appearances dead' after being carried up 34 fathoms (60 metres) from the bottom of the Scottish coal mine. Tossach describes how he: 'applied my mouth close to his, and blowed my breath as strong as I could'. But even before this published description, the Old Testament tells us how the prophet Elisha saved the life of a young boy by placing his mouth onto the mouth of the child.

The discovery of atmospheric oxygen temporarily halted the recommended technique of mouth-to-mouth due to concerns that exhaled breath was 'empty'. This is true to some extent, although the exhaled oxygen content of 16 per cent compared with atmospheric 21 per cent remains sufficient to resuscitate people during mouth-to-mouth ventilation. Nevertheless, due to these concerns the chest-pressure and chest-pressure arm-lift methods of artificial ventilation were developed, where pressing on the chest and even lifting the arms up above the head repeatedly was thought to induce artificial breathing. This comedic practice features in Arthur Conan Doyle's 'The Adventure of the Stockbroker's Clerk' where, after Holmes discovers a business owner hanging by the neck from his braces, Watson successfully performs the chest-pressure arm-lift, saving the man's life. The practice continued to be recommended until the 1960s when studies confirmed that chest compressions were more effective.

The 'C' component of CPR is the compression. I have pressed hard on countless people's chests, choosing the spot in the middle of the breastbone, where squeezing down 100 times per minute will allow the natural recoil of the ribcage to literally push and pull blood in and out of the heart. Doing this is both physically and emotionally tiring, never more so than during the prolonged episode of CPR I did on a three-year-old child as his mum held his hand and stroked his hair.

While the compressions of the heart between the breastbone at the front and the spine at the back squeezes blood out, the increased pressure in the pleural cavity compared with that outside of the lungs literally pulls blood out from the heart. Although external cardiac massage was first reported in 1892, it did not become accepted practice until 1958 when the colourful Brooklyn-born Dr William 'Wild Bill' Kouwenhoven combined it with his passion for electricity, allowing any abnormal heart rhythm to be reset using a defibrillator. This followed extensive work on resuscitation by Austrian doctor, Peter Safar, and an American, Dr James Elam. Like many medical innovations, this resuscitation technique was not widely adopted for more than fifteen years, despite evidence of its effectiveness. CPR evolved from being an invasive procedure in which the chest had to be surgically opened like a tin can, to the closed form of CPR used today.

Kouwenhoven's fascination with the effects of electricity on the human body was sparked by a spate of linemen dying in Brooklyn, New York, from an abnormal heart rhythm after receiving small electric shocks. He discovered that these deaths were due to abnormal patterns of cardiac electrical discharge, known as ventricular fibrillation or ventricular tachycardia – the same pattern the ambulance crew had detected in The Judge. Rather than heart chambers contracting in a neat sequence that allowed blood to be ejected, the cardiac muscle would frantically dance around in a useless fashion. Applying a DC current sufficient to reset this faulty wiring – yet not too high that it would damage the heart tissue itself – could revert a heart's rhythm back to normal.

Today, DC cardioversion can form a key part of resuscitation, along with external cardiac massage, when these abnormal heart rhythms are present. The widespread adoption of automated electric defibrillators (AEDs) allows the public to not only provide essential bystander external cardiac massage but also to apply electricity to these abnormal rhythms without danger to themselves or others. The self-contained machines automatically assess for the presence of deranged electrical signals, resetting them safely with a controlled electric shock. The Danish word given to this equipment, 'hjartstarter', gives a good description of its effects. These AEDs can even be delivered by drones in remote areas, allowing lives to be saved where the delay waiting for an ambulance to arrive would otherwise prove fatal.

Having learnt about these amazing resuscitation techniques,

why on earth would intensive care doctors not try to save the lives of everyone having a cardiac arrest? How could a DNAR order ever be a moral choice? There are two different scenarios in which a cardiac arrest occurs. The first is where a patient develops a primary problem with the heart or other organs that results in an unexpected arrest. This may be caused by a sudden heart attack, a clot on the lungs or even significant trauma. In these circumstances, we will do everything humanly possible to 'fix' the underlying problem leading to the cardiac arrest while performing CPR to give us the time needed to do so. The lengths to which we will go may even involve performing life-saving open-heart surgery at the side of the road, as one of my medical school colleagues in the Welsh air ambulance service did in 2017. French medical services have even put a patient having a cardiac arrest onto a portable heart-bypass machine in the middle of the Louvre in Paris while the *Mona Lisa* silently looked on.

The alternative scenario is when a cardiac arrest occurs in a patient with an already present and severe underlying disease that has reached its terminal conclusion. People with chronic heart disease, lung disease and terminal cancer will all die *with* a cardiac arrest. They do not die *from* a cardiac arrest. They die from their original disease, with a mode of death – the heart stopping – in common with all other human beings in history. In these circumstances, the cardiac arrest is a sign that the underlying disease cannot be fixed. Therefore, pressing on the heart will only result in the loss of dignity for the patient and emotional distress for the medical team doing the pressing. There is nothing that can be fixed and so any extra time CPR gives simply prolongs death rather than life.

Put in these terms, it is hard to understand why anyone would insist on having CPR during the sunset of their life. Most do not. People seldom take the opportunity to say 'no' through the application of a DNAR order. Why would they? There is little pleasure to be gained from having a conversation of this type with your loved ones outside the realm of imminent death, by which time it is often too late. I struggle to understand how people manage to have the degree of forward-planning needed to arrange a pre-paid funeral plan, and so it is no wonder that conversations about topics this emotionally charged seldom happen. That is perhaps why, as intensive care professionals, we sometimes need to lead the way and ask people for their views on these topics in a non-confrontational, open way. A distressing two-week patient admission to intensive care treating a futile prognosis is no surrogate for a difficult but honest conversation with a patient who has the right to make their own thoughts known. My palliative care colleague, Dr Mark Taubert, has advanced this public discussion in a remarkable way through both his 'Talk CPR' initiative, which encourages conversation about resuscitation for people affected by life-limiting illnesses, and his open letter published in the *British Medical Journal* in the wake of David Bowie's death, thanking the singer for helping others come to terms with death. This reads:

Oh no, don't say it's true – while realization of your death was sinking in during those grey, cold January days of 2016, many of us went on with our day jobs. At the beginning of that week I had a discussion with a hospital patient, facing the end of her life. We discussed your death and your music, and it got us talking about numerous weighty subjects, that are not always straight-forward to discuss with someone facing their demise. In fact, your story became a way for us to communicate openly about death, something many doctors and nurses struggle to introduce as a topic of conversation.

Now, please switch off your phone, close the door and put down your drink. It's up to you and me to transform this book from one that you read like any other, to a book that will potentially change your life and that of those around you.

If bystander CPR was performed consistently following cardiac arrest, on any given day thousands more lives could be saved. In other words, if you were to perform CPR on the next person you see having a cardiac arrest, they would be twice as likely to survive and return home following a cardiac arrest. And so that is what we are going to do. The best bit is, it's easy.

Take your right hand and simply place the hard heel part directly in the middle of your chest between your nipples. Now put your other hand on top. Next, get ready to sing. Press your hands up and down on your chest in time with the start of every word while repeatedly singing aloud the following lines from the Bee Gees' 1977 classic 'Stayin' Alive':

Ah, ha, ha, ha, stayin' alive, stayin' alive
Ah, ha, ha, ha, stayin' alive

You have just performed CPR in the correct position, pressing at just the right speed. Enrolling in a free CPR course will now make you even better. If you are ever aware of someone collapsing, not breathing properly and not showing any normal signs of life, you now have the skills to help save them. Ensure the emergency services have been contacted, get down on your knees and simply do what we have learnt. Keep your arms powerful and straight. Press down hard until you feel the chest move inwards. You will almost certainly not do harm but you may save that person's life. While there can be risks of doing CPR, not doing it carries the ultimate risk: a certain outcome of death.

Starting CPR early in cardiac arrest is critical to good outcomes. Even the fastest ambulance will not get to a patient and start CPR more quickly than you can standing next to them. Bystander CPR is always a good idea and I encourage everyone to get trained in its use and to do it. If you ever use this to save someone's life, please write to me and tell me. It will be the best letter I will have ever received.

~

We have learnt that starting CPR early is critical to survival. So too was the time taken to fix the abnormal electric pattern in The Judge's heart muscle. Knowing this, the paramedics quickly delivered up to 1,000 volts of electricity through The Judge's skin, which reached his heart and reset the frantic electrical chaos. While the CPR provided a temporary replacement for the pumping of the heart, this 'defibrillation' reset the electrical error and allowed the heart to pump for itself. The familiar 'mountain range' pattern returned to The Judge's heart monitor. Blood started once again to be pumped out, thanks to the team effort of the heart's four chambers being stimulated in the correct, sequential order. Life had returned. But, due to the length of time The Judge's brain had not received oxygen, he was put onto a life-support machine right there in the courtroom, as the press and the prisoner wondered what the future would hold. And I was now tasked with solving the life-or-death puzzle of what had caused The Judge's temporary death.

When I meet a patient who has had a cardiac arrest, I ask myself three questions: What has caused this? Can we fix it? What can we do to protect the brain?

There are a multitude of conditions that can lead to a cardiac arrest, although most frequently the cause lies in one of three main systems: the heart, the lungs and the brain (with the heart being the most common). Unlike what we experience in television dramas, with a character clutching their chest in pain, heart disease most commonly presents simply as sudden death.

Heart attacks are a form of heart disease where one of the three main blood vessels that supply the heart – the coronary arteries – becomes blocked. This obstacle consists of a mixture of clotted blood, fat molecules and hardened scar tissue from the vessel wall that has weakened over time before exploding inwards. When this blockage occurs suddenly, blood can no longer reach the heart muscle area supplied by that coronary artery. That part of the heart stops squeezing and can disrupt the normal electrical signals from getting to other parts of the heart.

Cardiac arrests can also occur even without a sudden blockage from a heart attack. Instead, scar tissue from chronic disease can cause sudden short-circuits that lead to abnormal heart rhythms such as the ventricular fibrillation seen in The Judge.

Major lung problems can also result in a cardiac arrest if the amount of oxygen transferred from the air to the blood is too low for the heart or brain to cope with. This may occur, for example, if a pulmonary embolus (a large blood clot) prevents blood from moving normally through the lungs. Finally, any number of brain catastrophes, including bleeds or strokes, can also wreak severe enough havoc on the heart to cause a cardiac arrest. Pressure on the brainstem from a bleed, or lack of oxygen from a stroke, can cause an outpouring of chemicals leading to very fast or very slow heart rates. The brainstem is also the 'control centre' of the body, regulating many essential functions including temperature, blood pressure and even how much urine is produced. Thus damage to areas close to this can quickly lead to physiological mayhem serious enough to cause a cardiac arrest.

When I sat down later with The Judge's family on the intensive care unit, I had a lot to tell them. It had been a busy night for us and for The Judge. I outlined how he had suffered from a cardiac arrest but, thanks to the swift actions of his colleague, he had reached hospital alive. We had already looked for the most common causes of this cardiac arrest. We had scanned his brain but found no bleeds or strokes. We had scanned his chest and found no blood clots, although a number of his ribs had been broken during resuscitation. (This was a good thing as it showed that the force of the CPR was sufficient to allow blood to get to his brain.) We had then taken The Judge to the heart lab, where a cardiologist placed a thin plastic tube, the width of a piece of dried spaghetti, through his radial artery in his left arm. This was navigated using X-rays all the way to the entrance of the coronary arteries that supplied his heart with blood. There we could see that there had been no new blockage of these vessels. He had not had a heart attack. There was evidence of more gradual narrowing of his arteries, likely due to a combination of age, diet and high blood pressure. These could not be treated with a balloon or a metal stent normally used to open up vessels blocked during a heart attack. Putting all of this information together, we concluded that accumulation of minor heart damage from years of low blood supply had caused fibrosis (scarring) in the electrical insulation of The Judge's heart's wiring, eventually causing his cardiac arrest. Sadly, that was when the trouble really started.

The first question I was asked by The Judge's wife during our initial meeting was the most common in these circumstances: 'When will he wake up?' This is also the question that we struggle the most to answer. I needed to explain that it was not a matter of 'when' but more a matter of 'if' he would wake up. Before exploring this, though, let's continue through the list of questions that I always ask myself. We had answered the first question (What has caused The Judge's cardiac arrest?) and so now – before we asked whether we could fix it – we needed to answer the next most pressing question: What can we do to protect his brain?

The evidence behind how to protect the brain is still uncertain at this time. There are studies showing that keeping the body at a cool four degrees below its normal temperature for twenty-four hours may reduce brain damage after a cardiac arrest. However, this may be the result of avoiding high fevers rather than due to the beneficial effects of targeting a low body temperature. We are currently conducting a large international clinical trial to help answer this very question.

We cooled The Judge down to a modest 36°C, keeping his body at this constant temperature for twenty-four hours by using a machine to circulate cooled water in plastic channels over the surface of his skin. We then waited another thirty-six hours for his body to slowly warm up and metabolise the drugs we had been using to keep him unconscious. If he survived this period, we could then try to wake him up. We would not know whether The Judge's brain had survived long enough for him to become conscious again until after this time. Unfortunately, The Judge's heart had other ideas.

The day after I spoke with The Judge's family, I returned to work hoping it had been a boring night. In intensive care, boring is good. Patients need time and stability, not excitement, to recover. Sadly, that night had been anything but boring for The Judge and the night team. Rather than settling down, The Judge's heart had entered a phase known as a ventricular fibrillation (VF) storm. This is a period of extreme and recurrent electrical chaos. One episode of VF, even when treated, simply results in another and then another. This becomes a self-fulfilling cycle where one cardiac arrest reduces the heart's blood supply, which then increases the chances of another arrest, and so on.

In the last twelve hours, The Judge had suffered over twenty episodes of cardiac arrest, requiring CPR and electrical resetting each time. It became so frequent that advanced procedures and treatments were needed. We had soon exhausted the shelf of drugs normally used in these circumstances. None had worked. Next, we tried inserting a pacemaker. This would artificially fire the correct patterns of electricity through electrical wires that ran through The Judge's veins to the inside of his heart. This didn't work either.

Finally, in the middle of the night, The Judge was taken back to the heart lab, where more tubes were inserted through his femoral artery at the top of his leg. These travelled up into the aorta. Around the outside of this tube was a sausage-shaped balloon, which we inflated over a hundred times per minute with low-density helium gas, allowing ultra-rapid inflation and deflation. This mechanically increased the pressure at the top of The Judge's heart where the blood entered his coronary arteries. Higher pressure leads to better blood flow, just like the water in your taps at home. Better blood flow hopefully would improve the function of the heart muscle and lessen the chances of further cardiac arrests.

By 6 a.m., the nurses and doctors drank their first cup of cold tea that night. The Judge's heart had succumbed to a period of grace. The Judge would not die that night.

~

We have explored two of the most common problems affecting the heart that I see in intensive care: abnormal rhythms and a lack of blood supply. Just like any muscle, the heart needs to squeeze correctly to perform its function and eject blood. Heart failure occurs when this ability is lost. This failure will come to us all one day. Nearly every mammal on earth, big and small, maintains a remarkable relationship between its average life expectancy and heart rate. This inverse relationship gifts mammals a billion heartbeats in their lifetime. For the hummingbird's heart, speeding along at over 1,200 beats per minute, this results in a lifespan of between just three and five years. By contrast, the blue whale's plod of just six heartbeats per minute is linked with an average life expectancy of over a hundred years. Humans have artificially inflated their number of lifetime heartbeats by increasing their age at death through improved lifestyles and nutrition. We now have around 3 billion heartbeats to use in a lifetime.

The severity of heart failure as a long-term condition is underestimated by professionals and the public alike. People living at home with even relatively mild forms of heart failure have a shorter life expectancy than some patients with cancer. This underlines the importance of the heart lying at the centre of our chest and at the centre of our health.

The last time you went to the gym, ran for the bus or even had sex, your heart needed to keep up. During a typical six-minute period of sexual intercourse ('typical' hides a wide variation, of course), your heart increases its number of beats from 400 to over 1,000. It does this to elevate the amount of blood being delivered to the rest of your body from 30 litres to over 120 litres. That is 160 bottles of the finest red wine. Alongside the increased frequency of beating, your heart squeezes much harder, ejecting 120 ml of blood every beat rather than its normal 80 ml.

While this may seem like hard work, it is nothing compared with the challenges that face any female partner present during those six minutes should it result in a pregnancy. Nine months after the initial excitement, the labouring mother-to-be will have a heart that is 10 per cent thicker than before. This extra thickness, due to muscle growth, will allow her to squeeze 50 per cent more blood out at every beat. Combined with lower pressure in her blood vessels to compete against, as much as 80 per cent more blood is pumped to mother and baby every minute during delivery. Amazingly, these physiological changes start developing from just five weeks into pregnancy.

At least this is what is meant to happen. A patient of mine called Lucy, and her baby, were not so fortunate. Being breathless during her daily walk wasn't new for Lucy. As a first-time mother with just three weeks until her due date, she had the nursery at home ready, lists of baby names carefully written and the method for collapsing the buggy honed to perfection. Lucy and her husband were prepared. But they were not prepared for their lives – and the life of their unborn baby – to be turned upside down so dramatically.

Any condition that impairs the ability of the heart muscle to squeeze will result in heart failure. The heart does not stop, it simply does not pump adequately for the needs of the body. If this occurs in the chambers on the right side of the heart, blood will pool in the body and the legs. Conditions affecting the left side of the heart will cause water on the lungs as blood is backed up and not pushed out. Wet lungs, like wet flour sticking in a sieve, do not allow oxygen to pass across their tiny holes into the bloodstream. Breathing is hard and ineffective. When both sides of the heart are involved, just staying alive is a struggle.

As she approached her due date, Lucy had to stop her daily walks. Her breathing was difficult even when at rest. Sleeping was no longer restful but hard work. Her ankles were the width of her arms, with fluid escalating up as high as her knees. Reading endless internet forums, Lucy became concerned about a number of conditions. She worried she had developed pre-eclampsia, a disease that often causes swollen ankles, breathlessness and high blood pressure. However, her blood pressure had been low over the last few weeks. Other mums posted that their breathing was also tough and their ankles similarly swollen. Perhaps, she wondered, this was just how pregnancy was meant to be? After a restless night sleeping upright in a chair, even walking to the toilet was impossible. Then Lucy collapsed.

Chronic health conditions, including high blood pressure, obesity, smoking and ischemic heart disease, account for over 90 per cent of cases of heart failure. Treating this is difficult and, as in all areas of medicine, prevention is better than cure. However, a number of drugs and devices have been developed that aim to improve the symptoms and outcomes for patients with heart failure.

When I meet a critically ill patient who is young, fit, and has no other medical issues, heart failure is a very unlikely cause of their decline. However, in the ICU, we admit the sickest of patients, which results in a skewed distribution of diseases. Walk around my unit today and you would be forgiven for thinking that brain bleeds, severe tuberculosis, leukaemia and patients with kidney transplants are common. They are not, but when they do occur, these patients often come to us. We don't see the masses who visit their family doctor with treatable conditions that get better. We see the one person out of a thousand who has a serious, rare problem that doesn't go away without treatment. We hear hooves in the distance and expect zebras not horses.

When I met Lucy, she was sweaty, her cold hands as blue as a bruise, and she had very low blood pressure. Her lungs were filled with fluid, her baby struggling to survive. She had all the signs you would expect with severe heart failure, but she was young and had no previous health problems. The tracing of her heart was abnormal in all parts, not just the areas supplied by certain blood vessels as would be expected during a heart attack. Using ultrasound techniques that just a week earlier had been used to show Lucy her baby, we looked at her heart as it struggled to squeeze. The right side was weak, the left side even weaker. She had severe heart failure with no obvious cause that we could find. We systematically thought of unusual causes: drugs or supplements she might have taken, hormonal abnormalities, vitamin deficiencies or problems with her coronary arteries that she may have been born with. Nothing fitted. The only remaining cause was the very thing that was most precious to her.

We have seen the extreme challenges that pregnancies pose even in healthy hearts adapting to the needs of a baby.

Rarely, pregnancy itself can affect the heart and lead to heart failure. Medicine loves complex terms and this one is no different. Called peripartum cardiomyopathy, this simply describes a problem with the heart muscle (cardiomyopathy) occurring around the time of pregnancy (peripartum). Although we still do not fully understand the causes of this condition, viral infections and abnormal immune reactions are the most likely contenders.

Consider alone the remarkable immunological feat of storing a baby – 3 kg of foreign material – within our bodies for nine months. The fact that this normally causes so few problems is remarkable. The ability to live with a fully formed human being inside you, drawing on your blood supply, is one of the most transcendent achievements of evolution. The roots of this ability lie in the gradual integration of foreign viral genetic code, as a side effect of common viral infections, throughout the course of mammalian evolution. A viral infection survives by 'hacking' into our genetic code, exploiting our cellular DNA machinery to produce millions of copies of itself. Even when common viral infections are cleared, fragments of their genetic code are left behind and woven seamlessly into our own genes, like empty boxes in the cellar. Most of the time these boxes simply take up space, but occasionally they become very useful. One such box contains the virus's ability to hide from our immune system during its replication phase. Like an undercover agent, viruses – including the common cold – can trick our body into seeing them as one of us and therefore into allowing them to use our body for their own purposes. This genetic ability was retained in the DNA of our distant animal evolutionary ancestors for reasons we do not understand, unused for millions of years until it found a new purpose: it now allows a human baby to hide from its mother's own immune system as humans exploit this ancient viral strategy to sustain new life. It is ironic that viral infections have both fostered this ability as well as resulted in so much heartache throughout the centuries by causing damaging congenital infections and – as most likely in Lucy's case – peripartum cardiomyopathy.

As Lucy's bed came through the automatic doors into the ICU, we were worried. In times of stress, going back to basics is often helpful. We try to concentrate on the three things that matter: giving a diagnosis, supporting the organs and treating the cause. Sadly, the diagnosis we were left with, peripartum cardiomyopathy, had no known treatment other than time or a new heart. We were therefore left with no course of action but to support Lucy's organs.

The normal treatments used when the heart cannot squeeze are powerful drugs that work on the cardiac muscle and blood vessels called inotropes and vasopressors. Inotropes increase the strength of heart contraction either by increasing calcium levels inside cardiac muscle cells or by sensitising the heart to calcium. Adrenaline, the ultimate inotrope, is found naturally in the body but can be delivered externally using pumps set to infuse at different speeds. Vasopressors literally press the vascular system, squeezing the veins and arteries. This not only increases the blood pressure but also helps to return blood to the heart from which it is then ejected again. The most common vasopressor is noradrenaline, a naturally occurring compound that we now produce synthetically.

Most critically ill patients will receive one or more of these drugs, delivered by tall banks of flashing pumps, blinking as they push their contents through thin plastic pipes. The drugs travel into the body through the large vessel in your neck, the internal jugular vein, or the leg's femoral vein. We measure their effects second by second, by watching the dancing trace of the blood pressure using tubes attached to an electrical transducer inserted into an artery in the leg or arm.

In Lucy's case it was clear that drugs alone would not suffice. Her hands and feet were cold, her kidneys had stopped making urine and her gut had stopped working. Due to her failing heart, she now had multi-organ failure. Although the drugs were encouraging her heart to beat, the demands of her body could not be met. Neither could the demand of her baby. As her organs began to fail, the trace of her baby's heart began to show signs of distress. It would record slow heart rates followed by periods of rapid beating at over 300 times a minute. To save Lucy, we needed to save her baby. So mum and baby were taken to the operating theatre together for an emergency Caesarean section. They would return separately. The little girl they called Hope was weak and floppy as she was cradled by the neonatal team. She would stay on a life-support machine just like her mum.

Although the demands placed on Lucy's heart were reduced following the birth of her baby, this wasn't enough. She continued to show signs of worsening heart failure, with her liver becoming enlarged from high pressure building up in the blood vessels connecting it to her failing heart. At first, we hoped the insertion of a balloon pump – the same device that had supported The Judge's heart – would help. While this did assist her left side in squeezing, it didn't help the fluid on her lungs or the right side of her heart. The next step was to give Lucy a new heart, but for now this would have to be one made of metal.

Medicine has had a long-standing fascination with the heart since William Harvey first described it as 'the circuit of the blood' in 1628. It is the most beautiful pump, soft, responsive to changing demands and perfectly rhythmic. The challenges of replacing its functions have still not been solved, although we now have mechanical support devices small enough to be implanted under the skin. These can sustain life – even in those with almost no heart function – for years. New developments now make it possible to live completely devoid of a heart. The former Czech firefighter, Jakub Halik, was the second patient to live without a heart, its function replaced by two implanted mechanical pumps. During the six months that he lived with a plastic heart, Jakub was even able to visit a gym despite having no pulse.

In Lucy's case, although offering her a heart transplant

was an obvious option, this was problematic. Finding a good tissue match before she died would be difficult. With a severe shortage of available donor hearts, the average wait on a transplant list is nearly three years. For Lucy even a wait of hours would be too long.

Huge progress in genetic engineering has been made since the first monkey-to-human heart transplant was performed in 1964, when the patient died after just two hours. (In fact, this was the first heart transplant performed in humans.) It is likely that organs from other animals – xenotransplantation – will be successfully transplanted into humans in the near future. However, most experts believe that this is still two to five years away and likely to start with kidney transplants between genetically engineered pigs and humans.

Even if a heart were available for Lucy, performing an operation in these circumstances would be difficult. There is a misconception that an organ transplant is the end of a patient's troubles. Transplantation is not a single inter-vention. Following any transplant, there follows a lifelong commitment to take powerful drugs that shatter your immune system, can lead to severe infections and even rare types of cancer. But with the potential for gradual recovery of heart function following delivery of Lucy's baby, we could give her the time she needed to recover without a transplant.

The first operation on a human using a heart-bypass machine was in 1951, although the patient died shortly afterwards. Two years later, in 1953 at the Thomas Jefferson

University Hospital in Philadelphia, an eighteen-year-old woman survived after having a hole in her heart closed using an 'Iron Heart' machine. These machines, although simple in theory, are extremely complex in both engineering terms and operation. They drain blood from the venous system, add oxygen to that blood before returning it, under pressure, into the arteries. The challenge lies in not damaging the delicate blood cells during this violent process while simultaneously preventing large blood clots. Using drugs to thin the blood needs to be balanced against the high risks of bleeding from the large tubes inserted into blood vessels.

With time, the size, complexity and costs of these machines have been reduced. We now have devices that are portable and able to replace the heart's function using only two large pipes inserted into blood vessels through the skin. This technology, known as extracorporeal membrane oxygenation (ECMO), uses gentle centrifugal pumps that protect blood cells while adding oxygen using an amazingly thin membrane with a large surface area. Bonding drugs to the inside lining of the machine's pipes reduces the amount of blood-thinning drugs needed, which reduces the risks of bleeding.

It was a hot Tuesday when Lucy was first put onto an ECMO machine. An ultrasound machine was used to guide pipes into her veins and arteries. Dark-red blood soon flowed through the clean, transparent bowels of the machine before it was expelled from the opposite side, bright red and full of life.

Take your index and middle fingers and place them

onto the side of your neck. Feel the *thud, thud, thud* of your heart as vibrations are transmitted up your aorta into your carotid artery. We did the same on Lucy's neck but, despite the ECMO machine replacing entirely the function of her failing heart, we felt nothing. The continuous flow of blood produced artificially would instead slip steadily into her body. She was alive but with no pulse.

The oxygen added by ECMO to Lucy's blood was high enough that just two days after her baby was born, Lucy awoke. The breathing machine was stopped, the tube in her windpipe removed and she could soon talk to us. The first two words she spoke were difficult to say and difficult to hear. She looked down towards her feet as her hand patted the flat bedsheets covering her tummy, and slowly asked: 'My baby?'

An hour after Lucy asked the most important question of her life, she would meet her daughter for the first time. Baby Hope's fight had been shorter than Lucy's, having spent just one night on a life-support machine in the neonatal ICU. As Hope's head pressed into Lucy's chest, she would not hear the heartbeat that had become so familiar to her over the last nine months. She would have to wait another five days before her mum's heart had recovered from its illness enough to squeeze by itself once again and she could be slowly weaned off the ECMO. Five weeks later, Lucy was caring for her daughter at home, ready to face the rest of their lives together.

~

At the entrance to my hospital is a domed area filled with shops, cafés, patients, relatives, hospital workers and occasionally pigeons. It is where news, good and bad, is broken between family members, where surgeons sit to discuss the complex cases of the day and where tired night-shift workers sip their overpriced coffees before journeying home. It is an area where a lot gets done.

After one particularly busy night shift, I was walking towards the automatic doors out of the hospital when a familiar face appeared. The Judge's wife had a spring in her step and a smile on her face. It had been nearly four months since I had met The Judge, and I worried that his wife still needed to visit him in hospital. I knew he had been well enough to leave intensive care, but the outlook for his brain was uncertain. Would he ever be able to recognise his family, feed himself, get home or even go back to work?

'He is so grateful for your team's hard work,' she told me. 'I've come to collect him after his operation. He is due back at work soon!'

I don't know whether it was a result of my post-night-shift emotions or the caffeine I'd consumed to get me through my cycle home, or both, but I felt a big lump in my throat. Here was a lady whom I had warned many times that her husband might not survive. Now their family could look to the future. The Judge was having a minor operation to fit a special pacemaker that would automatically deliver an electric shock should abnormal heart rhythms ever return. This would prevent the need for CPR and stop the vicious cycle of another heart storm from developing.

Weeks later I spent a few fascinating hours talking to The Judge and his wife about the dramatic events of his illness. The gravity of it had only sunk in when he saw spring trees blossoming through the window of the ambulance moving him to a nearby rehabilitation hospital. The last tree he had seen was bare, its winter branches creaking in the breeze. Now the trees had exploded with life and colour. The Judge had lost weeks of his life and his memory. This had a profound effect on his outlook and view of the future. He was reacquainted with the beauty of simple things once taken for granted. Being alive was sufficient to be happy. He had got back in touch with an old friend, had started going to the opera once again and was determined that work would no longer fill every crevice of his life. While in the rehabilitation hospital, he felt something unfamiliar since being a young boy at boarding school: he was homesick. The Judge was ready to leave – he *needed* to leave. After flying through his physiotherapy session that morning, he leant his crutch against the wall and walked without support for the first time. Then he climbed the flight of stairs that had been his nemesis for the last few days. Hours later he was at home, surrounded by cards from well-wishers, including one from the defendant in the original trial.

5

THE LUNGS

The open windows to the world

'I have seen many a man turn his gold into smoke, but you are the first who has turned smoke into gold.'

These were the words uttered by Queen Elizabeth I to Sir Walter Raleigh 400 years ago after he presented a strange new plant called tobacco to the English. That modern tobacco plant, *N. tabacum*, originated in the highland Andes, probably Bolivia or northern Argentina, in 6000 BC. As early as 5000 BC, tobacco was being smoked, chewed and even used as an enema by the Mayans as part of religious rituals. Christopher Columbus later discarded these tobacco leaves after arriving on the continent, and their utility was only recognised in 1492 by another explorer, Rodrigo de Jerez, after landing in Cuba. The cigarette, as we know it today, was introduced in 1830, when the South American *'papelate'* was popularised in France. Our relationship with smoking today has numerous parallels with the Mayans from the ancient past. It is almost a religion, certainly a ritual, or simply an escape from the humdrum of life.

Tobacco is the most dangerous plant in the world. Smoking it remains the leading cause of preventable death worldwide. It causes nearly 8 million deaths annually, 10 per cent of which are due to second-hand smoke. One in five deaths are tobacco-related, with smokers dying ten years earlier than non-smokers on average. In all, one-third of intensive care admissions, generating 40 per cent of costs, are related to substance misuse. Nearly 15 per cent of these substances are tobacco-related, compared with 9 per cent from alcohol and 5 per cent from illicit drugs.

A cigarette was the first thing after breakfast that would pass the lips of our next patient in the early neon blue of his Welsh mornings. It was Mervyn's escape from the brutality of his physically tough flour-mill job, and a source of relaxation at the end of a long, dusty day. Unlike the Mayans, Mervyn was able to smoke twenty times per day from the promising age of fourteen to the aching age of sixty-seven. When he started smoking it was not unusual or even discouraged. His mum worked in the local cigar factory and so smoking literally sustained the family. Just weeks after Mervyn had found the strength to lose his religion of smoking, I met him wheezing like an old church organ. I could hear him breathe before I could see him from the entrance of the hospital ward. He was as blue as his early mornings and about to die. Epidemiology told us why this was.

Epidemiology is the science of describing how often a disease occurs in different groups of people and why. This seemingly peripheral information can be used to spectacular effect, preventing further illness and hinting at the underlying causes of disease. Through applied epidemiology and public health measures, the lives of millions can be dramatically improved. This reach is far greater than any doctor treating individual patients even in a life devoted to clinical medicine.

The poster child of epidemiology is the London cholera outbreak of 1854, which centred around Broadwick Street in Soho. Today, you will find organic coffee shops and high-end fashion brands on this street, but the map that the English physician, John Snow, drew 160 years ago when examining the cause of this deadly cholera outbreak contained something far more telling. The clustering of cases around the water pump on Broadwick Street prompted him to examine a sample of the well's water under a microscope, finding that it contained 'white, flocculent particles'. Pre-empting acceptance of the germ theory of infection, Snow was convinced these flecks were the source of disease. After taking his findings to the parish leaders, they reluctantly agreed to remove the pump's handle as an experiment. Within weeks, the outbreak that claimed 616 lives was finally over. Incidentally, John Snow's remarkable achievements did not stop there. He later went on to safely use chloroform to assist in the birth of Queen Victoria's son Leopold in 1854, a turning point in the public acceptance of anaesthesia.

The British Doctors' Study published in 1956 was land-mark research pioneering a new epidemiological technique and gave conclusive evidence that smoking caused lung cancer. It was a new type of prospective (rather than ret-rospective) study, following 40,000 British doctors over fifty years from 1951 to 2001 in order to determine which environmental factors led to lung cancer and heart disease. This new statistical method was established by Sir William Richard Doll, a British physiologist turned world-chang-ing epidemiologist. His conclusions showed a doubling in the risk of death in smokers from both lung cancer and heart disease. There was no longer any doubt that cigarette smoking directly caused these conditions. We now know that many lung diseases we treat in intensive care – includ-ing infection, cancer, blockages, bleeding, asthma and air around the lungs – can be caused or worsened directly by smoking.

As you place that papery cigarette between your lips, you inhale 4,000 chemicals, of which forty-three are known to cause cancer, with an additional 400 poisons rushing down your delicate air passages. The nicotine will immediately cause your blood vessels to contract, restricting the supply of blood, which can cause a heart attack right then and there. Bible-black tar coats your air sacs as carbon monoxide gas prevents oxygen from being taken up by your blood. Formaldehyde – normally used to pickle dead bodies – combines with ammonia, hydrogen cyanide, arsenic and rat poison to cause direct tissue damage to the supporting structures of your lungs. This hacks into the building blocks of life, causing errors in your DNA. Each breath kills you and kills those around you.

Even if you do not develop lung cancer or vascular disease, the hot smoke and its poisonous passengers can lead to chronic lung disease. Chronic obstructive pulmonary disease (COPD) most commonly results from smoking (although industrial dust exposure and even genetic disease can also contribute) and affects one in twenty people over forty years old. Every cigarette smoked increases the amount of thick mucus produced by the passages in the lungs in a desperate attempt to protect themselves from harmful chemicals. At the same time, the tiny cilia hairs that normally sweep particulate matter up and out towards your mouth malfunction. This leads to accumulation of thick, dirty mucus, unable to escape from the lungs without forcible, red-faced, repeated coughing. At the same time, the spongy supporting structures of the lungs, which allow them to inflate and deflate efficiently, get eroded. Like an old elastic band found at the bottom of a drawer, they lose their spring and become weak. Air-trapping then occurs as the effort needed for each breath in and out increases. Areas of the lungs collapse, causing lower oxygen levels in the blood, while other areas remain blown up like an overinflated balloon. Your lungs crumble from an efficient, slick means of turning air into breath into an old, grumbling machine in need of replacement.

When I first set eyes on Mervyn, he could have been a

photograph in a textbook about COPD. Even a snatched glimpse of a patient from the end of the bed can reveal a myriad of secrets. Smoking combined with his years of working with heavy industrial dusts and diesel fumes had left its toll on his lungs. At the end of every breath, Mervyn would purse his lips in a desperate attempt to make each gasp last as long as he possibly could. This was not done consciously, but had a sound pathophysiological basis – the disease was affecting the physiology of his body. At the end of exhalation, your lungs reach a balance between the elastic recoil pulling inwards and your attached ribcage springing outwards. This leaves a surprising volume of air inside your lungs at the end of each breath.

Breathe out now to your normal level of exhalation before stopping. Next, forcibly try to blow out as much extra air as you can. You should manage around an additional litre. Even after this point there is another litre of air still inside your lungs. These additional volumes are called your function residual capacity (FRC). They play a critical role in maintaining a normal level of oxygen in your blood and keep your lungs at just the right level of inflation to make the work of breathing efficient.

Think back to the last time you blew up a balloon for a party. It would have felt tough when you first started to blow into that flattened promise of celebration. Similarly, as the balloon approached its size limit, inflating it further would have been hard. There was a sweet spot in the middle where blowing it up was easy. Your lungs work in a similar fashion. Mervyn's destruction of his elastic lung tissue had made his lungs very inefficient to inflate. Some areas of Mervyn's lungs were overinflated, some underinflated. They no longer had that sweet spot. Inflating a few tough balloons may be acceptable, but breathing 500 million times across a lifespan of eighty years causes considerably more problems. In addition, Mervyn's altered FRC reduced the oxygen reserves that could be used in times of crisis. Pursed-lip breathing was his body's last-ditch attempt at keeping his scarred, weakened airways open for as long as possible before they collapsed under the weight of fifty years of smoking.

Mervyn's neck muscles were large, powerful and strong. This was not due to his physical paid work; instead, years of 'enforced labour' from his lung disease had made them grow larger as the effort required to breathe had increased. They gave a helping hand to his diaphragm and chest muscles to just get through a normal 'healthy' day where he needed to breathe more than 20,000 times. Mervyn sat forwards in his hospital bed, his arms spread either side of his legs like a camera tripod as his body tried to assume the best position for maximising the power transmitted to his lungs, helping them to open and close over forty times per minute instead of the normal ten. His chest was large and barrel-shaped as a result of the air trapped inside. His fingers had lost the nicotine's saffron colour since he had stopped smoking. Instead, the ends of his nails now curled around his fingertips as extra tissue growth resulted from years of low blood oxygen levels. His ankles had become swollen from the high pressure in the right side of his heart needed to force blood through small, thick blood vessels, collapsed from the changes in his lungs.

From my initial, split-second impression of Mervyn, I knew he had severe COPD. What I didn't know was why it had suddenly become so much worse. Nor did I know if he would live long enough to see his family, who had been called urgently to the hospital.

~

Compounding the health reasons not to smoke comes the biggest shocker of all. Picture the scene. You have smoked for years. Despite the health effects, smoking brings you great pleasure. It's 3 p.m. on a Monday at work. You've had a hellish day, are feeling stressed, anxious and desperately in need of respite. Walking towards that quiet spot outside the office, you light up your cigarette or turn on your e-cig before inhaling deeply. As you exhale, a white cloud of smoke fills the cold air as your anxieties start to lift. You quickly feel calmer and better able to face the rest of the day. Put like this, who could argue that smoking doesn't have advantages as well as its disadvantages?

Sadly, this is all a cruel illusion and you are lying to yourself twenty times per day. What you experienced was more than a bad day at the office. Your stress and anxiety were actually your body's physiological response to nicotine withdrawal. The receptors in your brain had been trained over months and years to expect a level of nicotine stimulation equivalent to twenty cigarettes per day. In between these episodes, the lack of nicotine quickly prompts symptoms of acute drug withdrawal. The short-term solution is to satisfy this disequilibrium with an additional hit of nicotine. As soon as this happens, your body returns to its status quo, your 'normal' that has been redefined through habitual smoking. Your 'normal' is not really normal, however. Smoking that cigarette didn't make you relax, it simply treated an acute drug withdrawal that had made you stressed in the first place. You have simply returned to the standard level of function experienced by non-smokers every minute of every day.

The next time a cigarette touches your lips, think about that. Each cigarette is treating drug withdrawal, not delivering something extra. If you smoke, seek help and stop. Millions have already done this. Your friends and family have done it. You can do it too. Don't decide to do it tomorrow or next week or in the New Year. There is no such thing as a 'good time' to stop, but there is never a bad time.

Pick up your phone, send a message to your mum, your dad or your children. Tell them you are going to stop smoking. Put it on Facebook, tweet me, or write your pledge in the box opposite. Don't be that person who quits after being admitted to intensive care. Don't quit the day before your funeral. Don't leave this box empty. I don't want to meet you at 3 a.m. on a life-support machine. I don't want to tell your family that you have died because of smoking.

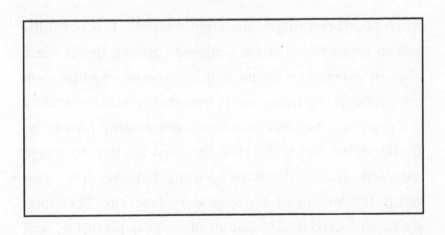

We rushed Mervyn towards the intensive care unit, with thoughts of what we could and should do. Supporting his lungs with machines might give us time to work out what was wrong and then to treat it. Seeing the exhausting work involved in breathing and the high level of carbon dioxide in his blood, we needed to help Mervyn take every breath. Although using invasive mechanical ventilation through a tracheal tube was possible, there were alternatives. These included non-invasive ventilation (NIV), an extra boost of air blown in from the outside using a tight-fitting mask, which allows us to adjust the amount of pressure given during each breath and provide additional oxygen. In COPD, this type of lung support can prevent the need for a life-support machine and improve a patient's chances of survival. NIV can also be used in the community to improve quality of life in patients with chronic respiratory disease and even severe sleep apnoea.

Imagine how it feels to have a firm plastic mask tightly strapped to your face. Now imagine having this done when your breathing is already impossible. It is not difficult to appreciate that for confused patients, this is not a pleasant experience. Some will feel a sense of suffocation even though the treatment is intended to achieve exactly the opposite. As Mervyn's illness was causing him to be confused, we had to balance the need for him to accept the mask against the risks of using sedative drugs that would further impair his respiratory function. Therefore, we administered small amounts of the drug ketamine, well known in the dance-party scene for its dissociative effects. Although ketamine can produce a deep sense of calm when used by trained professionals, it also maintains a patient's respiratory drive. When used by untrained amateurs in a nightclub, however, it can cause fitting, heart attacks, vomiting and kidney damage.

Ten minutes of NIV had decreased the level of carbon dioxide in Mervyn's blood, increasing the pH and improving his confusion. Examining his chest X-ray, we saw no fluffy white areas that would suggest infection and no air in the wrong places. His blood tests showed normal levels of infection cells and a heart tracing was also normal. It appeared that Mervyn had a non-infectious flare-up of his COPD, a condition that can occur multiple times per year in those with this disease. Any one of these episodes could be the patient's last.

Having made a diagnosis, we directed treatment against the abnormalities present in COPD. We added drugs to block the nerve receptors (called beta receptors) in the tiny muscles around Mervyn's airways to reduce air resistance. These drugs are inhaled by millions of asthmatic people every day using a characteristic blue inhaler. We also used potent steroids to reduce airway inflammation, and other drugs that break apart the protein structure of mucus to clear blockages from Mervyn's tiny air passages. Sadly, things did not improve. We then added a powerful drug that deactivates a key enzyme, phosphodiesterase, helping to relax airway muscles. You probably drink a similar drug yourself most mornings: caffeine is a naturally occurring phosphodiesterase inhibitor that can be used in rural locations without medical facilities to help treat tight lungs. Chewing instant coffee may not be a pleasant experience but it can help save a life in people with severe asthma and no access to help. For Mervyn, this new caffeine-like drug helped and finally his tight lungs became much looser.

Despite this initial improvement, however, Mervyn deteriorated once again a short time later. This time, no matter how much extra support we gave him using the non-invasive machine, it didn't help and so there was little choice other than putting Mervyn onto a life-support machine. As we prepared the tubes, the equipment and the drugs, I heard his family arriving behind me. Mervyn's wife and niece had arrived just in time. After I had spoken to them, we put the drugs, the equipment and the tubes away. Even though Mervyn was going to die without a life-support machine, we didn't use it. Why not?

I had initially thought that if we supported Mervyn's

lungs with machines we would have time to work out what was wrong and then we could treat it. But this was wrong. We shouldn't treat 'it'. We should treat 'him'. We should treat Mervyn. It is helpful to question who is the boss in an ICU. It is not the doctors, the nurses or even the relatives. It is not the hospital manager and it is not the judge in the medical courts. The boss is the patient. When they are critically ill, patients rarely have the capacity to consider or communicate their wishes. Therefore, relatives are often the best conduit to discover what the patient would have felt. Mervyn's wife and niece described to me in beautiful, tragic detail how Mervyn's lung disease had slowly chipped away at his life over the last few years. He had withered from a strong, powerful, confident man to someone who could not even walk out of his own house.

It can be hard to imagine that patients have another life before and after their critical illness. Caring for Mervyn at such a vulnerable time, I would never have guessed at his fascinating past. For years, his life was dedicated to the pursuit of health perfection. He had been a successful amateur bodybuilder for a decade, and his friends would call him a 'freak' as he effortlessly hurled around heavy bags of flour in the local factory. Years previously, Mervyn had been a top athlete, once beating a rival in a swimming race just two years before that person won bronze at the Olympics. He had also been a fantastic musician in his youth, a passion he would be forced to rediscover through disease. Predicting the breathless future stretching in front of him, Mervyn told his family he would not want to live should life get any tougher. He would not want to be resuscitated and would not want to be on a life-support machine. All Mervyn wanted was to stay well enough to indulge his remaining passions in life.

Bodybuilding had long been impossible since his diagnosis with COPD. He moved from sculpting his body to instead sculpting wood, and woodworking had become a huge part of his life. On one occasion, Mervyn had spent months carving away by hand at hard, American tulip-wood and maple to make a beautiful rocking horse called Megan, named after his dog that had died. Then, when his lungs could no longer muster the breath required to work this wood, he moved on again. Mervyn's cherry-red 1965 Hofner Verithin guitar had travelled to hundreds of clubs in the 1960s when his voice was loud and melodic. As the lead guitarist and vocalist in a four-piece band, Mervyn had played alongside the greats. Sadly his guitar had been lost in the 1970s but a secret plan by his wife to find and restore the guitar had come just in time one cold Christmas as his breathing was getting worse. The scratched surface hadn't been played for more than forty years, but within weeks Mervyn had fallen back in love with making his own music. This grew into a passion that kept life worth living.

The night after we had packed away the drugs and equipment needed to put Mervyn onto a life-support machine, I returned home and told my family about him. I had walked into the hospital the following morning with a predetermined sense of sadness, expecting a hollow space where Mervyn had been battling for his life. We had given him all of the drugs and treatments that might help his condition. Although we could not reverse his chronic lung disease, there was a small chance we could get him through an exacerbation just one more time. Sadly, by the early hours of the morning, things were not looking good. Mervyn's oxygen levels were dangerously low and his carbon dioxide levels dangerously high. Nothing was working.

Yet, as the night ebbed into dawn, things changed. Perhaps it was the steroids starting to work, perhaps it was the physiotherapy he had received, perhaps something else. Slowly, Mervyn started to get better. As I walked onto the unit that morning, his eyes were open, his wife was holding his hand and he asked for a cup of tea.

When I visited him a few months later back in his home, Mervyn looked like a different person. Yes, he was still breathless when he stood to greet me, but he was in control. Scattered around the house was evidence of his lung condition: multiple inhalers of different colours and a rescue pack of steroids should another exacerbation creep up on him. Mervyn had spent four days in intensive care needing NIV and a total of two weeks in hospital. He knew that before long, his lung disease would strike again. But not today. Instead, as I drank my tea, Mervyn sat in his favourite chair and explained how he was due to attend a rehabilitation course next week. He was determined that the six-week exercise programme would allow him to walk 50 metres without stopping, something he hadn't done for years. As he spoke, I noticed that he was missing a finger on his right hand, a result of an old industrial accident.

'I can't read music and I don't have all of my fingers any more,' he told me. 'So I just needed to invent my own way of playing the guitar again.'

As I clumsily strummed on his Gibson Les Paul, Mervyn picked up a beautiful handmade acoustic six-string guitar. His fingers weaved effortlessly between the strings as he played an almost perfect rendition of Eric Clapton's 'Tears in Heaven'.

'Do you want to learn? I know you're busy as a doctor but let me teach you,' he said.

I couldn't believe what I was seeing and hearing. This is why being a doctor is an amazing job. It's not the machines, the pay or the pension. It's people. People like Mervyn. We had given him back what he had most wanted. Time to live life on his own terms. This had only been possible because we had listened to his wishes. Intensive care can do a lot. But it should do only what is right and what patients want.

~

Between 2011 and 2015, I worked regular night shifts in a small ICU in Llandough Hospital. The hospital started life in 1912 as a specialist respiratory hospital, treating all conditions of the lungs from cancer to tuberculosis. The hospital also played an important, early part in developing medical research as we shall come to see. Its function has morphed continuously over time from a war hospital caring for prisoners to its most recent incarnation as a mental health unit, but it is remembered by many for its kilometre-long main corridor adorned by a painting of its history. Running to cardiac arrests for three years down its arrow-straight path certainly kept me fit, although it was a long, lonely walk back to the on-call room if the patient died.

When the night shifts were quiet, I had time the next morning to grow sepsis immune cells in a nearby laboratory as part of my research. Thanks to the time spent there, I completed my PhD. Medical research still plays a large part in my life, and I now help to run clinical trials into conditions as diverse as cardiac arrest, sepsis and nutrition along with a fantastic team of research nurses and my colleague Dr Matt Wise.

Medicine has come a long way over the last 250 years. In the past, clinical practices were informed only by unscientific anecdotes. Thanks to a doctor who also worked at Llandough Hospital, Archie Cochrane, this is no longer the case. Archie was the forefather of an epidemiological revolution during the 1970s, promoting randomised control trials (RCTs) as the best method to conduct medical research. Today we strive to use this research design to help direct which treatments we should be using, on which patients and at what time. RCTs bring scientific and methodological rigour to how we find out answers to tricky questions. They divide patients into two groups, giving the 'real' test treatment to one group, while treating the other with a 'placebo' (although some trials compare two active drugs to discover which one is best). Which patients get which treatment is random and the trial is conducted blindly so that neither the patients nor those caring for them know which treatment is which. The results are analysed using powerful statistical techniques that allow any bias to be removed, so that investigators can say with confidence whether a therapy works.

This trial design is considered the most robust and reliable. However, when I step onto my ICU tomorrow, 90 per cent of what I do will not be based upon this level of evidence. I am not unique in this respect. Many of the things that doctors do on a daily basis are simply a relic of circumstance or tradition. Although we endeavour to do what is likely to be best for patients, without further research we often do not know for sure whether this is the case. Tomorrow I will examine all of my patients with my hands and my stethoscope but, surprisingly, there are few studies to support these as useful practices. If the stethoscope were to be invented today, it would most likely not meet the current standards needed for approval of a medical device. Yet they continue to be used due to tradition, culture and a feeling that research studies are not the only arbitrator of what is best.

Even with practices that are based on some evidence, that evidence is often weak or, at best, prone to significant bias. Not all trial designs are as robust as the RCT. While it seems obvious, for example, that we should use antibiotics to treat all severe infections (as we do currently and certainly should continue to do for now), the evidence behind this is not hugely strong. It is based on looking backwards in time at previous groups of patients who did or did not receive antibiotics by chance. Following up on these patients over time, we see that the group who received antibiotics were more likely to survive. However, without using stringent trial methods including randomisation this could have been because they were looked after by a better team of people, may have been less ill to start with or had less underlying disease. In other words, while more people in the antibiotic group may have survived in these retrospective studies, this may not have been directly due to the antibiotics. The antibiotics could simply be a surrogate measure for other factors. These are known as co-founders.

To give another example, your chances of developing heart disease may be significantly higher if you read newspaper A compared with newspaper B. This is not because of the newspapers directly, but rather because those who read newspaper A are more likely to smoke, be obese, be older and have other unmeasured co-founders compared with the readers of newspaper B. This is why striving for high-quality research-trial designs, such as RCTs that remove unmeasured co-founders, is so important.

The lack of high-quality evidence in some areas is recognised within the medical community. It is not through lack of effort to change that we sometimes find ourselves practising blindly, but simply due to the complexity, costs and ethical issues surrounding clinical trials. Research now needs to move to the centre not the periphery of intensive care medicine and be strongly supported by government. The ethics behind clinical trials need to be explained to the public, and more research staff need to be properly trained and recruited. But this can be difficult to justify when staring at the immediate needs of a health system under strain.

As winter time approaches, I have a heightened sense of anticipation. How bad will this year be? How many patients will be critically ill with flu? Have my children had their vaccinations? Later, even as the Christmas adverts fade and Easter eggs start to appear on the shelves, hospitals remain full to the brim with the aftershocks of winter maladies. The 'Winter Crisis' is now simply 'The Crisis' as countless newspaper articles report. So why, as rotas remain under-staffed for the number of patients, do I sit in my office planning research studies? Why am I not out there working alongside my colleagues instead of running intensive care clinical trials? Why is scarce money being spent on placebo sugar pills that do nothing?

Some think that under such pressurised conditions, medical research is simply a nice added extra, only to be explored when the system is already performing well. They would be wrong. Research matters to patients, staff, and to healthcare. This is particularly the case in intensive care medicine where as few as one in ten of our treatments are based on the highest quality evidence. The rest may be ineffective, wasteful or may even cause unanticipated harm. Yet, the impact of an extra intensive care nurse is far easier to quantify than that same nurse working on a medical trial that will result in better care for countless future patients.

If you take part in a clinical trial, you are more likely to survive even if you only receive the placebo. If you are treated in a hospital that does research, you too are more likely to live than to die. The environments that nurture good research are also more likely to have good communication between staff, fewer vacancies and higher job satisfaction. Bringing the heads of different hospital experts together in a collaborative way can stop them from banging together in conflict. Washing hands and teaching others form core parts of working in a hospital. So too should research. It is the scaffolding onto which we can safely climb to search for better ways to help patients. Research may be the most effective pill we have.

Yet there remains a tension between money spent on research and that spent on 'frontline' healthcare, public awareness campaigns and quality-improvement measures. Some universities founded specifically to advance knowledge see research as simply 'money in, money out' when compared with lucrative post-graduate courses. Government campaigns rightly shout loudly about improving public awareness in areas such as early cancer diagnosis and recognition of sepsis. However, doctors can only do so much if they are not armed with treatments and diagnostics that actually work.

In 1999, 190 tragic deaths were caused by meningococcal disease in the UK. Fast forward to 2016 and just ten cases have been reported. You could mistakenly attribute this decline purely to the high profile media campaign showing parents how to identify the meningococcal rash using a glass tumbler pressed onto a skin rash. Yet the reality is that it was the hard graft of research teams producing a safe, effective vaccine, gained through expensive and time-consuming research, that also contributed greatly to saving those lives. Research matters.

However, advancing medical care through research focused on critically ill patients is difficult. The high rates of death and adverse events alone lead to a huge governance burden in clinical-trial reporting. The timings of admissions to intensive care do not follow a planned, predictable workflow schedule. One-third of patients are admitted after daylight hours and so, without a 24-hour research service, patients will miss out on recruitment into clinical trials. Furthermore, standard ways of asking patients for their permission to be involved in clinical trials are not appropriate in the most severely ill and unconscious. For example, a major international clinical trial in our unit examines the best temperature to use when cooling patients like The Judge following a cardiac arrest. This cooling period must be started rapidly within hours of the patient arriving, often late at night. These patients will be deeply unconscious, without capacity and hence unable to consent to take part in the trial. Alternative options, such as approaching a family member for consent (or, more correctly, *assent*), may be wholly unethical if they had been the one just doing CPR on their dad. This well-intended thought may simply add to their distress in a time of high crisis. Furthermore, needing a decision in such a limited timeframe would seldom be sufficient for truly informed consent.

And so what should we do? Should we simply continue giving treatments based on poor-quality evidence? Should we just keep our fingers crossed that these treatments are doing more good than harm? This would be unacceptable for those such as cancer patients, who have hugely benefited from research over the last fifty years. Similarly, this laissez-faire attitude and failure to engage with hard problems is not good enough for patients at their most ill and most vulnerable.

The use of deferred consent has helped to combat this research inequality. In trials without prior consent, after extensive ethical and legal scrutiny, patients can start to be given treatments before consent is given. The family will be approached for assent (approval) at the earliest appropriate time but not while reeling from the shock of sudden bad news. Here the family help us gauge what the view of the patient would have been had they been able to make the decision themselves. Should the patient recover, they too will be asked for consent to continue in the trial.

Conducting research without prospective consent raises concerns that it reduces personal choice and so erodes individual autonomy. Yet it is essential under certain circumstances, so as to answer important research questions, avoid potentially harmful delays in treatment of the very sick and prevent burdening anxious family members. Trials using this approach have already had a real, tangible and prolonged positive effect on the care of the sickest patients all around the world.

Even when we conduct high-quality research trials, some argue that the very system by which results are debated, selected and disseminated is inherently wrong. Medicine is stuck in the past. Today a clinical trial is conducted, the results calculated and a scientific article is written. For this then to be disseminated, it needs to be published by one of a small number of journals, each with its own tastes, motivations and ties to the pharmaceutical industry. It is estimated that over half of all studies are never completed and data from one-third of trials not published. Of those that are, only half are read by more than just two people. Furthermore, journals are more likely to publish papers with positive results, conducted by well-known groups, by men and from Western countries. This introduces yet more bias, known as publication bias. So, we now have bias squared. It is on this flimsy basis that we decide how to treat patients.

This selective publishing should not be acceptable in medicine. The former editor of the *British Medical Journal* has argued that the entire medical journal industry should be disbanded. The powerful 'all trials' movement led by Dr Ben Goldacre aims to publicise these issues surrounding clinical-trial data loss, manipulation and concealment. Times are (slowly) changing. One day I hope that medicine will use continuous improvement based on automated research techniques, applied for the benefit of all.

~

Helen and I didn't get off to the best start. Our first meeting ended with her shouting at me as I started my first night shift in Llandough Hospital near the coast of Cardiff. I completely deserved it. The ICU at Llandough was quiet and admitted few patients. I worried about getting little out of working in such a small place. I was very wrong. Spending time with patients like Helen taught me some of the most valuable lessons I would ever learn. One such lesson was the importance of communication when working as an intensive care doctor.

Effective teamwork uses the currency of communication to purchase trust, but the theatre of care is an extremely challenging environment for achieving this most basic of human needs. Communication is one of the riskiest things we do in medicine. Too often 'meant is not said, said is not heard, heard is not understood, understood is not done'. Even communicating simple gestures can be complex in hospital. It can be noisy, busy and stressful. Critical care teams are thrown together in the fog of an emergency, often having never met before. The late Dr Kate Granger was an inspirational British doctor who recognised this fact. Before sadly dying from cancer aged just thirty-four, she left a simple yet impactful legacy of insights she gained from being a patient herself. Having stood on both sides of the hospital curtain, she noted how few healthcare workers actually introduced themselves to her by name. Omission of this simple gesture is understandable in the furore of a busy hospital, yet for patients it can be devastating. Her campaign, 'Hello, my name is', reminded us all to use this simple gesture. This was my intention as I pulled back the curtain around Helen's bed area at the start of my first night shift. I popped my head through the opening and said: 'Hi there, I'm Matt, the new doctor.'

'Get out!' was the response hurtled towards me.

Helen was one of a small number of long-term patients on the ICU. She had been attached to a ventilator, all day and all night, for two years when I first met her. Although there are no robust statistics, it is thought that around 3,000 patients live in their own homes, needing a ventilator, in the UK. Helen's journey had started years previously as a passenger in a road traffic collision. A serious spinal injury meant that she was transformed from a healthy woman in her twenties into someone needing to use a wheelchair for the rest of her life. Tragically, a second collision years later caused yet more spinal damage. This was when I met her.

Our ability to breathe is dependent not simply on having healthy lungs. Although our delicate air sacs perform gas exchange, the physical act of sucking in air requires a functioning diaphragm, nerves and muscles. After Helen's second injury, her spinal cord could no longer transmit messages correctly to her diaphragm. These impulses normally run along nerves exiting through gaps in the third, fourth and fifth vertebrae near the top of the spine. Just below this level are the nerves operating the hands and arms. With Helen's spinal cord damaged at such a high point, she was not able to move her arms, hands, legs or even her diaphragm. She needed a machine to breathe for her.

Even though she was attached to a life-support machine, Helen's inner life was the same as it always had been. She could think clearly, see normally and hear normally. The things she loved and hated were the same. Communicating with her while attached to a ventilator was difficult. A tracheotomy was performed, partially to help communication but also in the hope of improving her strength enough to wean her from the ventilator.

For anyone attached to a ventilator, even for just one day, breathing independently again can be a challenge. Muscle wasting occurs just hours into a period of critical illness and, combined with an impaired cough, can be a significant barrier to successful weaning from mechanical ventilation. Just like running a marathon, breathing for yourself again may require significant physical training. Before starting any weaning regime, all underlying medical problems should first be treated as best they can. Like the first session with a personal trainer, we then explore any barriers to training. These may include a weak heart, too much sputum, excessive muscle weakness or poor nutrition. After this, the real work can start.

We started training Helen by gradually reducing the amount of help delivered through her life-support machine.

Each day, we dropped the extra boost in air pressure provided by the machine by as little as 1 cm/H_2O. After weeks of hard work, Helen's level of support needed to be increased once again. Her muscles were too weak, her cough was ineffective and her lungs were continually filling with thick mucus. We were taken back to the start line.

It is recognised that individuals differ in their responses to physical training techniques. An old friend of mine from medical school has applied the explosion in personal genomics to provide bespoke exercise programmes based upon your genetic blueprint. Through analysis of a saliva sample, his genetic-testing company can help predict whether high-intensity training is right for you. We are now working together to apply this disruptive technology, offering previously unaffordable genetic testing direct to patients preparing for the greatest challenge of their life: surviving critical illness.

Appreciating this variation, we tried a new weaning strategy for Helen consisting of short, sharp periods of removing almost all breathing support. These 'sprints' were initially possible for stretches of just a few minutes. Soon they were stretched out to periods of over one hour at a time. Sadly, as autumn turned to winter, Helen was no closer to the finish line and so we needed to change the type of race we were training for.

The reason Helen had shouted at me during our first meeting was because I had broken a cardinal rule. I had treated her not as a person but as a patient. If my regular postman opened my front door, climbed the staircase, pulled back my shower curtain and handed me a letter, I would shout at them too. That is essentially what I had done to Helen. The small ICU in Llandough was Helen's home. She had spent two years there, attached to a ventilator, while waiting for her new house to be built. By then it was clear that she would need a ventilator for the rest of her life. Helen couldn't finish the original 'race' for which she had been training so hard. Her body was never going to become strong enough to come completely off a ventilator despite her years of trying. So we changed the goal, changed the rules of the race, and instead hoped we could get Helen home safely. Victory would now mean striving for independence while needing to remain on a ventilator.

As I pulled back the curtain around Helen's bed without warning during her personal time, I took away her privacy and what control she retained over her life. I would never do this again and Helen and I quickly became great friends. We shared laughs and tough times. She would tease me about the brightness of my pink shirts and I would confide in her about aspects of my life shared with few others. I would often think about Helen during physically tough points in my life. I remember one summer struggling at the halfway point of a cross-country race. The one thought that kept my legs moving forwards was how much Helen would give to feel even a fraction as tired as I did from running. Sadly, just weeks before Helen's new house was ready, she died. It felt like a big piece of the ICU died with her.

~

Through recognition of the challenges in medical research and human thinking, we can now celebrate the fact that intensive care has never been such a safe, successful and cost-effective service. You are almost twice as likely to survive today from sepsis – the main reason for admissions to the ICU – than fifteen years ago. The chances of you getting home following a cardiac arrest in the community are 25 per cent better today than just a decade ago. We can put oxygen directly into a failing heart and keep someone with no lung function alive for over a month. We can allow surgeons to carry out operations inconceivable in the past, including heart and face transplants. Every day we look at patients' lungs using ultrasound, and place needles just a millimetre thick into blood vessels, organs and even into the brain. The world of intensive care is changing, just as the world of medicine is changing. The lungs will continue to be the open windows to the world but they need the fresh air of research and human-thinking improvements. Medicine is richer and patients better served as we embrace the benefits of these new research methods and insights into human critical thinking and we prioritise honest communication in difficult situations like those faced by Mervyn and Helen.

6

THE BRAIN

The ghost in the machine

When it comes to the line between what medicine can do compared with what medicine should do, I often face uncertainty when meeting elderly, frail patients with severe chronic disease who develop seemingly reversible conditions. While these problems may be fixable in the short term, their future impact on a patient's life is often not. The concept of survivorship – embracing the long-term impacts that critical illness leaves in its wake – is better appreciated by families than by some in my profession. A success in our eyes has too long been simply the state of being alive at hospital discharge. This is not what patients or their families would describe as a success. They instead want their story to conclude by returning to an independent, mobile and fulfilling mental and physical life. The patient wants to survive not just in a narrow sense, but in a broad sense, with an acceptable quality of life.

Predicting the outcome after a brain injury is fraught with uncertainty. On more than one occasion, I have been sent videos of past patients whose families were told the likelihood of a meaningful recovery was tiny. I watch with simultaneous joy and dismay when I see these 'patients' playing football or chess better than I do. Joy because we did the right thing for that patient. Dismay in case we have been overly pessimistic about other patients in the past.

I am equally affected by patients who survive but are left severely disabled. The impact of poor functional recovery after critical illness can destroy the family relationships, marriages, emotional well-being and financial security of those left facing the consequences of our 'success'. This is before even considering the devastating impact it can have on the patient. Is this an acceptable cost? I don't know.

~

Steven's partner held his hand in hers. It was warm and felt familiar. The colourful monitor above showed a perfect set of observations. His heart was beating strongly, sixty times per minute, his lungs were working well and all of his blood tests were normal. She could hardly believe that her partner, father to their five-month-old baby girl, had died an hour ago. How could this be? Just twelve hours earlier, Steven had been at work. The challenges of becoming a new dad were very real. Weeks of sleepless nights and end-less nappy changes had taken their toll. He was tired and had a throbbing headache. For many new parents trying to balance a busy working life and their home life, this will sound familiar.

Steven had earlier said goodbye to his daughter as her mum took her outside for some fresh air. That would be the last time that Steven's daughter would ever hear her father's voice. After returning home, Steven was found lying on the floor of the kitchen. Despite his partner's efforts, she could not wake him. When Steven was brought into the emergency department, he was deeply unconscious.

We use a graded scale to assess the level of a patient's alertness called the Glasgow Coma Scale (GCS). This scale was developed by Professor Jennett and his trainee Dr Teasdale (now Sir Graham) in 1974 at a world-leading brain-injury research centre in Glasgow. The GCS is still the most commonly employed way to communicate changes in a patient's level of consciousness. The lowest score out of a maximum of fifteen is reserved for patients who do not talk, do not open their eyes and do not move even when painful pressure is applied to the bone underneath the eyebrow. When we added Steven's scores together, he had the lowest possible of $1 + 1 + 1 = 3$. He was in a coma and we didn't know why.

A coma can result from a number of problems inside or outside of the brain. Outside, the common causes include effects of prescribed or illicit drugs, high levels of toxins from liver or kidney failure, low body temperatures, high levels of carbon dioxide from lung failure, and other salt imbalances. A basic panel of tests confirmed none of these was present in Steven.

Within the confines of the skull, a number of diseases cause coma. While seizures commonly result in repeated, violent movements, following a fit the brain has a period of shutdown called the postictal phase, from the Latin after the 'ictus', meaning a blow or strike. The patient will remain unconscious while in this phase as their brain struggles to recover from the extreme electrical storm of the fit. Other rare seizure types also cause unconsciousness without any movements occurring. Lack of blood supply to the brain due to blood vessels becoming blocked (ischemic strokes), especially those at the base of the brain, can also result in coma. A build-up of fluid on the brain, infection of this fluid or infection of the brain tissue itself can gradually cause a patient to slip into a coma.

The story of Steven's sudden collapse did not fit with any of these scenarios. A patient's story in medicine is as important as the tests we do. A diagnosis is only secure once the story, the tests and the patient all fit together like life's sudoku. When you work it out, it is like being let into the secret of an amazing magic trick, knowing the big reveal. Sometimes this never happens and, no matter how hard we try, the rows and columns of numbers just do not fit. In Steven's case we were worried that a spontaneous bleed had occurred in his brain, and sadly we would be left with a perfectly aligned grid of numbers: the story fitted, the scan of his head agreed and so did his clinical examination.

Our priority in the initial stages of caring for Steven was to reduce any further harm. Being unconscious in itself is not particularly dangerous. However, what can happen during unconsciousness can kill you. Think back to the last time you choked while drinking water or eating a crisp. The coughing fit that ensued was not taught to you by your mum or dad. From the moment you were born, the impulse to forcibly contract your diaphragm against partially closed vocal cords – coughing, in other words – came naturally to you. The evolutionary quirk of placing your food pipe immediately behind your breathing pipe could hardly be described as 'intelligent design'. However, it did allow your ancestors' vocal cords to rise high in their neck, increasing the ability to make new sounds. This literally gave us a voice and so, despite the increased risk of choking to death, the advantages outweighed the disadvantages.

When unconscious, the brain's stalk (the brainstem) is unable to initiate these automatic life-saving reactions. Combined with the stomach's impaired ability to empty its contents following a brain injury, Steven's clean lungs were in danger. You may have been told stories about someone so drunk that they vomited in their sleep and choked. The same thing can occur after an injury to the brain. We needed to protect Steven's lungs from this danger by intubating his trachea. Therefore, even if he did vomit, it would not get past his breathing pipe to damage his clean lungs. This would give us time to see whether Steven had a chance at surviving.

Although unconscious people have reduced cough reflexes, the process of tracheal intubation is still hugely stimulating: the vocal cords can react at any moment, causing difficulty in inserting the tube, and the lungs can be left too tight to be ventilated using a breathing machine. Therefore, we use powerful sedative drugs before intubation to deepen unconsciousness, along with drugs to prevent muscle contraction.

Michael Jackson is a testament to the effectiveness of our most commonly used sedative drug, propofol. Its 1976 discovery by Imperial Chemical Industries (ICI) in the UK revolutionised anaesthetics due to its safe, predictable and usually helpful effects. Like all drugs, propofol comes with a 'consumer information leaflet' in its packaging. However, it is a prescription-only drug and should be used only by those with appropriate training. Even if a nuclear reactor came with an illustrated step-by-step assembly guide, the very fact of needing this help would mean that you are unlikely to be the right person to put it together. When propofol was used by Dr Conrad Murray, the side effects of this white, milky emulsion led to the death of the world's greatest pop star.

When Dr Murray injected Jackson with propofol it led to the deep unconsciousness that the King of Pop so desired. But injecting the drug is the easy bit. Keeping the patient safe through constant monitoring is the critical next step, one that Dr Murray didn't provide. Instead, he left Jackson alone while he visited the toilet. Jackson didn't have the one-to-one expert at his bedside to ensure his breathing was adequate, neither did he have the skilled nurses there to carefully infuse the drug slowly into his veins to maintain just the right level of sedation required. Jackson was not in an ICU or operating room, perfectly designed to use the drug safely. Instead he was in a bedroom, alone, and, as a result, he died when his oxygen levels fell so low that it resulted in a cardiac arrest.

For Steven, paralytic agents formed the second mixer – alongside sedative drugs – in our cocktail to keep him safe. These are a fascinating group of drugs, purified from plant material by the Macusi Indians of Guyana, who named the plant extract curare. Originally employed to paralyse prey using drug-tipped blowdarts, these drug molecules fit like a key into a muscle's lock. They fill perfectly the gap in protein receptors designed for the neurotransmitter acetylcholine at the junction where nerves connect to skeletal muscle. The drug blocks these receptors from receiving correct signals, therefore preventing all voluntary muscle contraction.

There have been rare occasions where paralysis drugs have been administered without the concurrent use of sedatives. This causes the terrifying syndrome of awareness under anaesthesia where patients remain unable to move, blink or scream but are entirely conscious during surgery. Thankfully, due to increased awareness, education and the use of monitors to indicate the level of consciousness during an operation, this is extremely rare. You are far more likely to get hit by a bus on your way to hospital than to experience this rare phenomenon after arriving.

Once Steven's lungs were protected by using these drugs to insert a plastic tube into his windpipe, we moved him to the safety of the ICU. When the final report of his brain scan came through, his future played out in my head like an old movie I had seen a hundred times before. He had developed a massive haemorrhage from a large, ruptured blood vessel at the front of his brain. These dilated areas of blood vessels, or aneurysms, can occur in 5 per cent of people due to a combination of unlucky genetic inheritance, high blood pressure and other lifestyle factors including smoking. Only a tiny minority of these will ever burst; we just can't predict which ones.

Bleeding from the delicate blood vessels that supply the brain can cause a brain injury. The bleeding in Steven was from an artery in the front of his brain that had ruptured and caused blood to accumulate between the innermost layers where spinal fluid normally bathes. This is called a subarachnoid haemorrhage, a bleed underneath (sub) the arachnoid (spider-like) layer surrounding the brain.

Bleeding between the next layer, underneath the tough connective tissue of the dura, is called a subdural haemorrhage. This layer contains thin-walled veins rather than arteries. Bleeds here often occur in patients taking blood-thinning medications and in alcoholics with smaller, shrunken brains. I remember vividly an elderly, homeless lady who was brought into hospital presumed to be drunk and asleep. It turned out she had suffered a large subdural bleed.

Moving up another layer, our brains have a space between the skull and the outer brain's surface where larger arteries run. This is the extra (outside) dural space. Bleeds here happen when sharp, bony spikes rip and pierce through the thick arterial walls following a fractured skull. Having a crowbar connect at high speed with one's skull is an effective means of causing this type of bleed. There are also bleeds that occur in the brain tissue itself, called intra-parenchymal haemorrhages, often occurring from sudden deceleration forces in restrained car accident victims or else without warning in patients with high blood pressure.

Occasionally we will care for someone after a road traffic accident who, despite having no evidence of bleeding on a brain scan, remains deeply unconscious. Sadly, the images we see when looking at brain scans are only a pictorial representation of the brain. The complexity and intricate nature of the organ that makes you a person cannot simply be represented using pixels of light. These pictures do not tell us the full story about a brain's correct function. When extreme forces of acceleration or deceleration occur in high-speed accidents, the connections between nerves can be destroyed, along with the stretching of nerve fibres. This injury, called a diffuse axonal injury, is difficult to appreciate on a normal scan, although more in-depth magnetic resonance imaging (MRI) scans can sometimes reveal this hidden damage.

The bright white appearance of blood on Steven's scan was filling almost half of his head and blocking the small exit channels where his spinal fluid normally travelled down to the bottom of his spinal cord. Without an exit route for this fluid, the pressure in his brain was extreme, preventing blood from moving through the base of the skull. There was already evidence that the bottom of his brain was trying desperately to find a way to relieve this pressure by squeezing through small bony holes at the bottom of his skull, and this was causing more damage to the brainstem, the part of the brain essential for life.

While operations can help some patients with this condition, sadly for Steven it was too late. Nothing could have prevented him from collapsing that day; it was only a matter of time with an aneurysm so large. Had it not happened then, it would have been the next day or the day after that. From the moment his bleed occurred, Steven would not have been aware of his future or have suffered any pain. This was the only solace we could give to his young family as they waited anxiously in our relatives' room.

Doctors deal with countless tragic situations such as Steven's. It is no wonder, therefore, that a commonly asked question from the public is: 'How do you deal with this?' For me, the line between work and life is so blurred that it provides little in the way of separation. Working with people during the most intimate, painful parts of their lives affects me deeply and for ever. This creeps into even seemingly insignificant parts of my life. I cannot wear a shirt any more without rolling up the sleeves. We do this routinely in intensive care to reduce infection.

In a deeper way, I struggle to be compassionate towards friends and family who tell me about their relatively minor injuries. These pale into insignificance compared with what I deal with day in, day out. Unless you are unconscious or not breathing, I have little to offer practically or emotionally. At the same time, I am unreasonably squeamish when asked to deal with my children's minor injuries just hours after having my hands deep inside someone's bleeding chest cavity. There is no line between the roles in my life yet a deep one all at once.

We shall return to Steven's journey later in the book. We will explore what it means to be alive and what it means to die. For some, death is not the end of their role on this earth; it can be a new start in a strange way. For Steven, our care for him and his family did not stop when he died. We continued to care for him for twenty-four hours after death, and care for Steven still continues in one sense to this day.

~

Joe's story is sadly familiar. He was a typical teenager who was admitted to hospital late on a Saturday night following a violent fight. He had a passion for winning. Every weekend Joe would fight, sometimes four different people, punching them hard in the face and body. Sometimes his parents would be only metres away. Occasionally he would get injured, sometimes knocked out. But this didn't faze him. As soon as school came on Monday morning, he would look forward to next weekend's fight. Yet Joe had always been a calm-natured boy, polite and helpful. Why would he act like this? Why does anyone?

Think back to the last time you spent time in the waiting room of an emergency department. You may have experienced shame when reflecting on the stories surrounding you.

To your left was a drunk man with a bloodied nose after an alcohol-fuelled fight over his favourite sports team. To your right were the immediate, distressing effects of domestic violence. Hidden were the long-term costs to those people's lives and the lives of others: a criminal record leading to unemployment, or broken relationships and children left without loving parents. A single foolish mistake. This is my plea to you, your friends and your family: even a single, foolish punch harms. Occasionally it kills. Walking away does not.

But this wasn't Joe. He was never drunk, never broke the law and had a lot of love to give. He was a rising star in the world of amateur boxing when he was brought unconscious to the ICU as an emergency.

It hadn't been a good day for Joe. His first boxing opponent had dealt him three strong blows in a row during the first round. Each time, his head would buckle backwards as his brain floated in the protective sea of spinal fluid produced by the ventricles. Like jostling ice cubes in a glass of whisky, Joe's brain would strike the frontal area inside of his skull after each punch. Millions more delicate neuronal connections were destroyed each time than would have resulted from drinking that whisky.

His second opponent delivered a body blow low on his diaphragm, causing Joe to gasp for breath as the bell thankfully sounded. By opponent number three, Joe was tired and dazed. Just ten seconds before the hammer was due to hit the wooden plinth in the third round, signalling the end of the fight, the periphery of Joe's vision faded to headache grey. His young body crumpled to the mat as his bloodshot eyes closed. They wouldn't open again for two weeks.

As I approached Joe's bed in the white light of intensive care, there were all the telltale signs of what had happened. The book *Blink* by my hero, Malcolm Gladwell, beautifully describes the human brain's immense ability to make accurate judgements from tiny snippets of information. (This was based on the work of Nobel Prize winner Daniel Kahneman and his late colleague Amos Tversky.) From simply a brief glance towards Joe's bed, his problems were clear. Firstly, I could see the white propofol syringe slowly injecting its payload to keep him deeply unconscious. Next, I could see the ventilator fighting hard to keep Joe's carbon dioxide levels just right. The bank of flashing monitors included a characteristic wavy line with two distinct peaks representing the pressure inside Joe's head. Finally, he had a thin plastic tube inserted through a small drill hole into one of the lakes of his brain through which spinal fluid normally flows. These interventions were all designed to protect Joe's brain from further injury after we discovered a large extradural bleed resulting from that last flying fist.

The sedative drug propofol was reducing the amount of work his brain needed to perform. Less work meant less blood and oxygen required and so less potential for further damage. We kept his carbon dioxide levels normal using the ventilator to maintain the amount of blood going into and out of his brain. The balance of blood entering and leaving your brain is called cerebral perfusion. It is carefully balanced, with the setpoint dependent on a number of variables, but carbon dioxide levels – the same gas that makes your champagne fizz – are the most pressing in this scenario. Too low and not enough blood would flow to the brain, causing further damage through oxygen starvation; too high and Joe's brain would swell. Like your home's central-heating system needs its water flow, your brain needs a constant blood flow to stay warm. If the pressure in the brain builds up, we need to squeeze blood through arteries even harder to maintain the same flow. With Joe, we used the pressure monitor inserted into the brain tissue to help guide how much squeeze we needed to use. Every minute we were able to adjust his blood pressure using drugs to maintain this set flow. Although Joe didn't know it, the way we managed his brain injury had strong connections to a famous past resident of Cardiff.

~

One question I ask junior doctors during ward rounds is about the connections between Cardiff, *The BFG* and intensive care medicine. Surprisingly few know that the cathedral village of Llandaff, just a mile from our wards, was the home of the world's most famous children's writer, Roald Dahl, and that he was christened in the Norwegian church in the bay area of Cardiff, still visible to patients gazing through windows from the top floor of the hospital. Dahl left behind an important legacy promoting better treatment and prevention of critical illness that is often eclipsed by his literary success.

Although born into privilege, Dahl had a tough life interspersed with tragedies from the age of three when his sister died of sepsis from a ruptured appendix. Later, as a fighter pilot in the Second World War, he came close to death after landing his Gloster Gladiator biplane hard in the Egyptian desert and breaking his nose, fracturing his skull and being knocked unconscious. In the five years between 1960 and 1965, things got even tougher. First Dahl's three-month-old son, Theo, was hit by a taxi in New York and sustained a brain injury. Then, in 1962, a letter home from school warned the family of an escalating measles outbreak. There was no effective vaccination, so Dahl acquired a single dose of 'gamma globulin' for his son from the head of the Lister Institute of Preventive Medicine, who was married to Dahl's half-sister and who agreed to import this gamma globulin from America. With Theo still weak from his accident, this single dose of antibodies concentrated from donated blood, which can transiently prevent certain contagious diseases, was given to him. Three days later, Dahl's seven-year-old daughter Olivia came home covered in spots. Three days after that, while she was recovering, Olivia beat her father at a game of chess. The next day she was dead. Olivia had died because the measles virus had spread to her brain, inflaming the delicate, tissue-thin linings and causing encephalitis. To end this period of tragedy, Dahl's actress wife, Patricia Neal, was admitted to the intensive care unit after a large bleed from a brain aneurysm aged just thirty-nine while pregnant with their fifth child.

Dahl attacked each of these issues with tenacity and energy. His son's brain injury had caused 'water on the brain' (hydrocephalus) from blockages in the exit routes for brain fluid, experienced daily by patients with brain injuries in intensive care. Like a high-pressure plumbing problem, this fluid needs to be drained before it causes further brain damage. Despite pipes being inserted connecting Theo's brain fluid to his abdomen, they repeatedly became blocked. Since Dahl's flying accident, he had indulged his engineering passion by building model aeroplanes, and now he employed these skills to adapt an aircraft fuel-line design into a new valve that would prevent blockages in hydrocephalus. The Wade-Dahl-Till (WDT) valve was patented in 1962 after a collaboration between Dahl, the hydraulic engineer Stanley Wade and the neurosurgeon Kenneth Till. There are still people alive and walking around today with this little piece of the famous writer inside them.

Olivia's death from measles also helped countless others. *The BFG* was dedicated to Olivia, written fourteen years after the introduction of a vaccination for measles that would have saved her life. In 1986, four years after *The BFG* was published, Dahl made a passionate plea in a deeply personal letter encouraging the widespread adoption of vaccination to prevent others experiencing the pain of loss he endured. Public health authorities still use this letter in publicity campaigns today. It ends with the following words:

I dedicated two of my books to Olivia, the first was *James and the Giant Peach*. That was when she was still alive. The second was *The BFG*, dedicated to her memory after she had died from measles. You will see her name at the beginning of each of these books. And I know how happy she would be if only she could know that her death had helped to save a good deal of illness and death among other children.

It is tragic that 2013–18 has seen the rate of measles infections rise by over 300 per cent across Europe, matched by a failing immunisation rate due to misguided worries about vaccination safety. The successful vaccination programme against polio in countries around the world today prevents a repeat of Vivi's story every minute. Millions of children have been saved from a lifetime of disability. Yet, when diseases are less visible, it seems irrational fear around vaccination safety can grow, unfettered by the invisible yet larger rational worry about the actual disease.

Dahl, the medical pioneer, had one more campaign to wage. His wife's stroke in 1965, was treated initially with convalescence and just one hour of physiotherapy per day. This made little sense to Dahl: 'Surely one hour a day is not enough. What in the world are you going to teach a child if she only goes to school for an hour a day?' Dahl's wife struggled to move, struggled to eat, and her garbled voice inspired the Gobblefunk language in *The BFG*. She had a lot to learn. With the help of friends, Dahl designed an intensive six-hours-a-day regime. 'Slowly, insidiously and quite relentlessly' his wife recovered and even managed to resume her acting career, receiving an Oscar nomination for *The Subject Was Roses*, which was released just three years after her stroke. Patricia further developed these methods, which we still use in intensive care today, into a book that led to the formation of the Stroke Association. A writer can change the world, not just through words, but also through actions. I hoped that Joe would one day benefit from the rehabilitation techniques developed by Dahl and his wife, but first he would need to survive.

~

The day after I met Joe, I started a run of three night shifts. If you have a sense of impending doom on a Sunday night anticipating work the next day, night shifts are that same feeling but on fire. Sleeping during the day before is impossible for me; instead, I cram in those boring tasks that our busy family cannot normally find the time for. I bank cheques, wash the car and occasionally grout the shower. The life of a doctor is seldom like the off-duty antics in the TV show *ER*. I then spend the evening thinking of my 9.30 p.m. start. The dread of starting a night shift is quickly replaced by the pace of work, before a sense of sheer elation upon finishing thirteen hours later. I end my shifts with a good breakfast in a local café and a strong coffee for the drive home before I crawl into a fresh bed like an old sloth.

As I head into my forties, the link between sleep

deprivation and the brain is becoming increasingly clear. Some days I sleep at night, some days I am forced to be a day-sleeper. The ICU where I work is unusual, having a senior consultant resident in the hospital every hour of every day. If your mum is critically unwell at 3 a.m. on Christmas Day, she will still meet me or one of my colleagues regardless of the unsociable hour. While there is no guarantee that this immediate senior presence improves the chances of survival, it does allow the sickest patients to be seen within minutes by the most experienced doctors. It simultaneously allows difficult ethical discussions and decisions to be made in the middle of the night. Having a consultant 'on call' at home, tucked up in a warm bed, is a tremendous psychological barrier to having end-of-life conversations with relatives of sick patients who perhaps should receive palliative care on a ward instead of an admission to intensive care. In our system, these conversations happen night in and night out.

There are costs to pay for this way of working. While I could stay up all night during my twenties, I now long for immediate sleep as my night shift ends. I am grumpy in the daylight before a night shift starts, and I suffer from a sleep hangover for days afterwards. The fantastic book *Why We Sleep*, by the American neuroscientist Matthew Walker, beautifully translates these costs into human terms while explaining the science behind our essential slumber. He argues that lack of sufficient, quality sleep is more detrimental to health than the classic risk factors that family doctors aim to modify, such as obesity and hypertension. Night-shift workers in Denmark who developed breast cancer after years of working night shifts have even received compensation based on this evidence. Summarising the importance of rest, it terrifies me to admit that shorter sleep leads to a shorter life through increased risks of developing heart disease, obesity, dementia, diabetes and even cancer.

Even more problematic are the effects that night shifts in intensive care have on the risks you pose to others. This was illustrated devastatingly by the case of Lauren Connelly. After a tough six years studying medicine at Glasgow University, Lauren landed her ideal job working at a rural Scottish hospital. Seven weeks later, she was exhausted. After a run of busy day shifts, working nearly 100 hours per week, she started the first of her seven night shifts in a row. She would not finish these and instead died tragically on 17 September 2011 on Scotland's busiest motorway as she fell asleep at the wheel of her car.

As I drive home after my first shift in a run of nights, I am more dangerous than a drunk driver. My reactions are poor, my visual awareness blinkered and my emotions labile. Even if I manage to grab three hours' sleep at night, my chances of having a crash are nearly twelve times higher than someone who has slept for seven hours. Should I fall asleep at the wheel, unlike a drunk driver who brakes late, I am unlikely to brake at all: crashes involving tired drivers are far more likely to be fatal.

But now that we know these risks we can do something

about them. I now sleep before driving home after a busy night. I am selfish about sleeping between shifts, using eye masks and earplugs to block out the distractions of my family life. I check critical decisions at night with others and use checklists to offload my brain.

There has been a lot of public debate around the provision of rest facilities and improved conditions for doctors. Some feel that workers are paid to work, not to sleep. Others feel that doctors arguing for contractual change are motivated by money rather than time to do their job and to do it safely. I wonder whether knowing that long hours actually increase the risk of harm will persuade our leaders to embrace the lessons of the past. The stories of doctors working 100-hour weeks, often with little time for rest and recovery, should be a national scandal rather than a rite of passage. You would not step onto a plane with a tired, exhausted pilot with reaction times slower than a drunk driver. Neither should you step into a hospital under these same conditions, yet this happens every day.

Sleep deprivation is not restricted to the staff working on the ICU, however. Imagine that tonight you plan to sleep in an unfamiliar single bed, in the middle of a busy hospital ward, surrounded by equipment as noisy as industrial machinery. Every hour, a nurse you have never met will shine a bright light into both of your eyes. Every four hours, they will turn you from one side onto the other to prevent sores, while you wear a flimsy hospital gown that barely covers your dignity. While you 'sleep', a confused alcoholic patient just metres away starts screaming and swearing. On your other flank, a young girl who has been in a road traffic accident dies after the medical team tries in vain to resuscitate her. The sobs from her parents are not muted by the paper curtain around her bed. All the while, crisp neon lights are turned on and off as an endless melody of alarms chimes like birdsong. At 8 a.m. sharp, just as you manage to drift off, a young doctor wakes you up, shakes you by the hand and asks: 'Did you sleep well?'

Even if you have no illness and are given no drugs, intensive care is a dreadful place to sleep. It is a dreadful place to 'get better' in the broad sense when an illness is mild. You might have the worst cold in the world, but you would not want to recuperate with a Lemsip on an ICU. The consequences are more than an inconvenience even in the short term: just brief periods of insomnia have severe health effects. A single night of sleep deprivation impacts the body's temperature regulation, decreases insulin sensitivity, increases blood pressure and causes hallucinations accompanied by confusion. Considering that critical illness affects your circadian rhythm, and powerful sedative drugs destroy sleep cycles, it is no wonder that acute delirium is common on the ICU. Being cared for in intensive care is fantastic when you are very ill, but moving to a ward environment is just as important when you are better.

The word delirium was first used in medical writing by the second-century Greek philosopher Celsus to describe a temporary mental disorder during a fever or after a head injury. Today we use this term to describe disturbances in mental attention coupled with memory problems, disorientation or perceptual faults. The underlying scientific basis for delirium is still unclear, although imbalances of neurotransmitters in the brain including dopamine and acetylcholine – similar to the patterns seen in dementia and psychiatric diseases – show promise as the most likely explanation. It is no coincidence that lack of sleep disturbs the levels of these same neurotransmitters.

As I walk through an ICU, delirious patients are easy to spot. They look agitated, confused, scared, often reaching out towards things that are not really there. Delirious patients can punch, kick, swear, spit and are difficult to manage even for the most experienced nurse. These are the patients with hyperactive delirium. At the other end of the spectrum, those with hypoactive delirium shrink into themselves, not speaking, not interacting with others, but looking equally terrified. Both conditions are frightening for patients and relatives alike. When I first meet the family of a critically ill patient, I tell them to expect delirium as part of their relative's illness since up to 80 per cent of intensive care patients will experience it at some point. Far from simply being a scary phase to navigate through, delirium can have an enormous impact on the short- and long-term health of patients. Those with delirium spend more time on a life-support machine, more time in hospital, have a higher risk of developing dementia, and ultimately are more likely to die for reasons that are unclear.

Patients who have recovered from delirium can describe their terrifying delusions in high-definition detail. Some swear they were taken to an airport while unwell, with an endless parade of suitcase trolleys being wheeled backwards and forwards. Others say that dogs were licking and nibbling at their feet for days on end. These strange memories often have a real material basis, exaggerated and distorted by a delirious mind. The airport scene was in fact a patient whose bed was opposite the medical equipment room, with trolleys often used to cart suitcase-shaped boxes in and out. The licking dogs represented a machine strapped to the patient's legs and feet, squeezing up and down every few minutes to reduce the risk of blood clots. Listening to these delusions can help us to improve the environment that we sometimes take for granted.

Unfortunately, delirium is difficult to treat effectively. We lack a miracle cure and instead strive to prevent it or simply keep patients safe when they are delirious. This can be done by improving the environment to better orientate people along with providing good nursing care. Despite this, strong sedative or antipsychotic drugs are sometimes needed. An alternative but less palatable strategy is to use soft hand mittens or, in extreme cases, physical restraints. The decision to use these methods is not taken lightly. Doctors are one of the few professions with the legal powers to deprive people of their liberty, but they do so only under extreme conditions where all else has failed.

There is a positive message to take from all this. Huge improvements can be made to patient care even without expensive new drugs or complex technology. What we can do instead is recognise the importance of a good environment for sleep quality. Simplicity is best. Using sleep masks and earplugs, while striving to maintain day–night light cycles and reducing false alarms on the wards, can be effective. Single rooms allow those recovering from critical illness the physical and psychological space to get well. Reducing noise wherever possible is essential. Research from our unit led to the introduction of soft-close bins, preventing the clash of metal on metal hundreds of times per day. This nods to the importance of building design: ICUs should increasingly consider patient experience as a key factor in recovery, and the bricks and mortar of a hospital ward can affect this experience as much as the humans working within the walls.

As public health systems struggle to balance their finances, investing in the physical environment of a hospital is a particularly hard sell. Yet decades of research have shown that physical surroundings influence not only people's behaviour, but also their wellbeing. Broken lifts and draughty windows may quietly suggest that patient care is also at risk, yet proper investment can turn these whispers into loud voices of approval. One of the greatest improvements in my professional life was the renovation of our hospital canteen. Having well-cooked, healthy, hot food served in a nice environment goes a long way to improving morale.

Educating both patients and staff about the importance of sleep costs little but promises big returns. Research in this area – previously ignored – may give further insights into how sleep manipulation could impact on functional recovery. Together with early mobility (encouraging patients to move and get out of bed) and noise reduction, promoting good sleep can help prevent the temporary madness brought on by delirium.

~

When I arrived for my night shift, I was delighted to see that the pressure inside Joe's head was in the normal range of just 2–3 cm/H_2O. However, it steadily crept up over the course of my night shift as further patients arrived on the unit. When brain pressure increases despite our use of measures such as controlling the blood's carbon dioxide levels, it signals one of three things: there is a new mass inside the brain (often further bleeding), the patient is fitting, or the brain tissue itself is swelling. When the pressure increases to such an extent that blood struggles to flow in, something needs to be done. We decided to take Joe off the unit, still attached to a breathing machine, to do a further scan of his head in the middle of the night.

Transporting somebody while unconscious and critically ill on a life-support machine is not something we take lightly. There are risks in being moved; equipment can become dislodged and monitoring can fail. Even the act of physically moving people on the edge of life can tip them over the edge of physiological disturbance. But in some cases it is still essential to understanding the problem, as without finding problems, we have nothing to fix. It was worth the risks in Joe's case as his scan showed that, although there was no further bleeding, his brain was dangerously swollen. The decisions that followed were both simple and complex.

Theoretically, the simplest way to reduce the pressure on the brain is to remove it from the bony confines of the box in which it resides. It's not exactly brain surgery, but it is. Removing the skull top – a decompressive craniectomy – has been practised for more than 120 years. It reduces the pressure inside and hence improves blood flow to the brain. It should therefore result in better outcomes for patients. That would be the obvious conclusion. But beware of the obvious conclusion in medicine! Many treatments that have previously been considered beneficial have later been shown to cause overall harm – in critical care alone, this list is long. Transfusing blood to achieve a normal level of haemoglobin has been shown to cause more deaths. Giving high amounts of oxygen to people with bad lungs may cause more deaths. We have learnt over the last ten years that less can mean more, and so we no longer aim to achieve supra-maximal physiology (levels of organ function higher than normal) or even normal physiology; we aim instead for just enough.

Similarly, when applied to a broad range of patients with brain injuries, a decompressive craniectomy does produce more survivors, but with an increased likelihood of severe, profound disability overall. We cannot predict if the patient will be a survivor with a good outcome or a survivor with a very bad one. Statistics help populations of people but not individuals. Not only that, but all operations come with risks as well as benefits, and the decompressive craniectomy procedure is complex and fraught with dangers including bleeding, damage to the brain and infection. Nevertheless, in young Joe, we had little choice. Without the operation he was going to die. His parents felt Joe would accept the risks of profound disability in order to hope for the slim chance of a good outcome. He had the major operation while his parents paced up and down the corridor, not sleeping but simply hoping that their young boxer would be able to fight against the toughest opponent he would ever face.

But Joe's fight was not over after his life-saving brain surgery. Christopher's story demonstrated how infection can rage against the life of even the fit and young. Following major surgery, we often encounter problems quite removed from the original pathology. A brash surgeon may claim that 'the operation was a success, but the patient died'. The tirade of reactions our bodies mount after surgery mirrors that of our distant ancestors recovering from a vicious animal attack. The immune system fights to repair our tissues while it struggles to keep infection at bay. Our heart comes under additional stress and our guts enter hibernation. Stress hormones can lead to muscle breakdown and even kidney failure.

Joe's normal defence mechanisms were already impaired before his operation, after which his vulnerability to infection became an even greater challenge. Sometimes latent viral infections, such as chickenpox or the cold-sore virus, become reactivated. Other infections can attack the plastic lines inserted into veins, and developing pneumonia while on a breathing machine is common. Yet Joe had survived that first night after surgery. His brain pressure reduced, no bleeding occurred and the surgeons were happy with their results.

The second night shift of caring for Joe, we became concerned that he had developed a severe lung infection called ventilator-associated pneumonia. When patients are unconscious on breathing machines, the normal defence mechanisms that protect the lungs become impaired. The patient does not cough, their mucus is not swept out from the windpipe, and gel-like material produced by bacteria (a biofilm) forms around the plastic of breathing tubes. This creates a perfect environment for bacteria.

It can be difficult to distinguish lung infection from other causes of low oxygen levels in critically ill patients. We scanned Joe's chest, looking for characteristic shadows inside his blood vessels caused by blood clots, but there were none. Instead, we saw fluffy white areas where the lung's black air spaces normally are found, representing excess fluid in the air sacs. This fluid was most likely due to a new severe lung infection. Joe was soon receiving the maximum amount of oxygen our machines could deliver. Despite the antibiotics, he had developed septic shock, kidney failure and multi-organ failure. I spent hours talking with his mum and dad about our concerns. Our passion in life as critical care doctors is fixing problems that can be fixed. With Joe's young age and potentially reversible disease, we would not stop until it was fixed or became unfixable.

~

After three years at medical school, the endless dusty science books and sickly smell of the dissection hall had taken their toll. Just in time, I was given the chance to spend one year away from Wales to study for a degree in a subject allied to medicine. As a protest against the hours of cold molecular biochemistry I had endured, so removed from the warm ward patients, I applied to study medical law and ethics at Bristol University. This transported me away from the sterile, white laboratory into grand old yellowing buildings. I was immersed in classes with statute-quoting law students and philosophy students with beautiful, flowing handwriting. My ability to handwrite even a few short sentences had been amputated during medical school and I found the going tough. After a term of studying ancient English medical law and Kantian discourse, I felt more adrift than ever. I struggled to superimpose the endless two-dimensional pages of text onto my three-dimensional patients. Fifteen years later, and I now apply the principles and lessons I learnt during my time in Bristol each day when treating real, three-dimensional, critically ill patients. The scholars studying medical law and ethics, developing paradigms for withdrawing life support from critically ill patients, are doing important theoretical work that truly touches the lives of many, albeit from a safe distance. Meanwhile, it is our privilege, burden and responsibility as critical care doctors to apply these laws and theories while looking into the distraught eyes of the family.

The tough decisions I face on a daily basis are often reflected in the tragic stories told in the media of children with critical illnesses whose lives hang by the thread of a court decision. Parents and doctors can find themselves in irreparable conflict over what is the best and just way to treat someone they both care for. These decisions, as complex and as hard as they are, can be reduced to one simple question: What is in that patient's best interests?

For me to insert tubes into your veins and place your body onto a life-support machine, I need your consent. Your ability to provide this consent first requires you to have the 'capacity' to be able to do so. Before asking for consent to take a sample of your blood with a needle, I must be satisfied by several preconditions: you must be able to understand why a blood sample is needed; you must appreciate the risks involved as well as be able to independently weigh and balance these risks against any benefits; finally, you must be able to communicate your thoughts back to me. This process seems rather long-winded for an act as simple as taking a blood sample. Were you to be offered a heart transplant, these factors would suddenly become much more salient. Only after you are deemed to have capacity would any decision be possible through valid, informed consent.

When I met Joe, he was deeply unconscious and critically

ill and would not have been able to fulfil any of these tests of capacity. Therefore, how could I do any of the things needed to save his life without his consent? No other person can consent on behalf of another adult without prior legal powers being in place, and so doctors must often rely on an alternative strategy when patients lack capacity. Instead of seeking patient consent, we act according to that person's best interests. In Joe's case, it was clear that being a fit, young person facing critical illness, he would have consented to interventions that would save his life had he had capacity. I judged in an instant that it was in Joe's best interests to be placed on a life support machine and have tubes inserted to save his life.

Two weeks later, after the storm of sepsis and multi-organ failure had blown away, we were faced with another decision affecting Joe. After surviving his severe brain injury and multiple infections, we were unable to safely take Joe off the ventilator. He was still in a coma and without a tracheotomy he would not be able to survive independently. His breathing was too shallow and his cough too weak. The implications for this procedure were profound. This is not due to the dangers of a tracheotomy directly but because having one can allow people with devastating brain injuries to survive additional weeks, months or years. Although a tracheotomy may allow Joe to survive, this may be accompanied with severe physical disability. He may have remained dependant on others for washing, moving, feeding and going to the toilet for the rest of his life. Joe lacked the capacity to decide for himself, being unable to communicate, unable to appraise the risks and benefits, and hence unable to consent to this procedure. In this scenario, whether a tracheotomy was in Joe's best interests or not was far from clear.

It is often assumed that family or a patient's next of kin 'decide' to 'turn off the life-support machine'. This is not true in most critical care practice. Instead, a patient's family play a crucial role, not as decision-makers, but as advocates for their loved one who cannot speak for themselves. Although I had known Joe for weeks, his parents had known him for sixteen years. They were better placed than I was to consider what Joe would have wanted in the scenario that he faced. Although this doesn't form the entire basis for a best-interest decision, it is of immense importance. His parents told me that Joe was a fighter in life and that he would remain a fighter when facing death. So long as there was a chance at a life with some independence, Joe was the sort of person who would grasp at that tightly. These factors, combined with the potential for recovery, helped form a best-interest decision. We felt that it was in his best interests to have a tracheotomy. His parents agreed and so life and Joe and treatment went on.

The high-profile cases featured in newspapers often tell the other side of this story. They mostly centre around tragic cases where a patient's best interests cannot be agreed between the healthcare team and the family. In cases where the brain injury is so severe that the patient has no chance of a meaningful recovery, continuing treatment may not be in the patient's best interests – regardless of the family's hopes. Instead, symptomatic treatment focused around the alleviation of suffering may be a better focus. In these cases, remaining on a mechanical ventilator would no longer be treating a reversible problem but instead would simply cause further discomfort. Therefore, withdrawing the ventilator and allowing nature to take its course is aimed not at precipitating death but at alleviating distress from treatments no longer in a patient's best interests. I often phrase this when speaking to families as: 'We will continue to use all the treatments that may help, but we will not use the treatments that will not.'

Ultimately, the conclusion of withdrawal of treatment in intensive care is often death. Some families may never accept that this route is the right one. The doctor who has spent days, weeks or months aiming to save life – but whose actions now result in death – can find their halo slips to a noose when viewed through family grief. When faced with these conflicts, what should families and critical care doctors do? What is right and just for the patients who cannot speak for themselves?

The first strategy must be formed around allowing time, compassion, understanding and communication. These issues are hard – and should be hard because they involve people who care. Most of the time, these simple elements of humanity are enough to precipitate what is best for the patient we all care about. In the tiny minority of cases where this is not enough, the unhappy direction of travel is increasingly to the courtroom for a prolonged, expensive and painful process resulting in the announcement of a best-interest decision on the patient's behalf. With the increasing medicalisation of terminal disease, accompanied by a more rapid advancement of what we *can* do compared with developments in what we *should* do, I fear this trend is set to continue.

Anyone with capacity is perfectly entitled to make decisions that are strange, misguided, foolish or even downright stupid. A good friend of mine has a passion in life that I regard as being firmly on this continuum: on a sunny Saturday afternoon in rural Wales, Mike will voluntarily climb aboard an aeroplane, ascend to 5,000 metres and then – with only a thin nylon parachute to prevent his death – throw himself out of its side door. Although strange to me, Mike has the capacity to make any foolish decision in his life including skydiving. Similarly, in hospital, patients are perfectly entitled to decline treatment, even when this decision will result in severe harm to them or even in their death. Therefore, so long as capacity is present, I will continue to honour the decision of any Jehovah's Witness who is at liberty to decline a blood transfusion even if it means a completely preventable death. While this feels like a grave, illogical and foolish decision, I am not them just as I am not my friend Mike.

~

When I arrived at Joe's home a year and a half after his injury, his presence could be felt as soon as the front door swung open. Now living permanently back in his family home, the effect of his brain injury on his parents was clear. They were tired yet happy, injecting all of their energy into coming to terms with a new 'normal' for them and their son. In the lounge, following me with his blue eyes, were photographs of Joe pictured at the peak of his fitness. Wearing gold medals around his neck like a town's mayor, he looked strong, happy and determined. As I turned my head, there was another person looking at me. He too was strong, happy and determined.

Joe had survived his walk across the bridge between life and death. He had spent over six weeks unconscious in intensive care – first with a severe brain injury, then recovering from his major brain operation. Severe pneumonia had necessitated a prolonged period of mechanical ventilation using a life-support machine. When his oxygen levels had dipped so low that they were incompatible with life, we used a different machine that breathed more than 300 times per minute. He had battled multi-organ failure, needed kidney dialysis and had survived early liver failure. Minute by minute, we had pulled Joe through his illness and he had held on tightly. We need not have worried about the long-term impact his severe illness would have on his life and that of those around him.

'Hi, Dr Matt!' Joe said in an almost musical Welsh tone. He had a sparkle in his eyes and was keen to show me how the left side of his body was regaining strength. He was sharp, his language excellent and his mood good. The scar of his tracheotomy was barely visible, covered by the collar on his T-shirt, and his voice was strong. The injury being on the right side of Joe's brain was fortunate. If you are right-handed like Joe, the parts of your brain important for language (Broca's area and Wernicke's area) are located in your left brain. These were thankfully spared from direct injury. Extensive rehabilitation had allowed Joe to make huge leaps towards a life where he could look after himself, manage everyday activities and plan for the future. He told me how he had met with his opponent from that final boxing bout. Rather than resentment and anger, the meeting led to forgiveness and friendship, ending when Joe gave him a silver St Christopher, the patron saint of travel, as a parting gift. Joe's journey has just started. As he turns nineteen, he has enrolled to study computer science in his local college. The light in his eyes has continued to burn bright.

7

THE GUTS

The fire in your belly

When I think back to my holiday in the scorching Croatian heat, I picture myself sipping my new favourite cocktail, the negroni. Thought to have been created in Florence by the Italian Count Camillo Negroni in 1919, it is a stiff drink combining one part gin, one part vermouth and one part Campari. Remembering that holiday scene today fills me with pleasure: I can recall the creative yet subdued hue produced by the cocktail. Yet I simultaneously dread the harm alcohol has done – and continues to do – to patients, their families and the fabric of society. Along with tobacco, alcohol is by far the most dangerous recreational drug that we encounter in intensive care. This is due to its widespread use, the chronic and acute effects it brings, and the propensity to cause its users to act as fools. It damages individuals and they damage others. That negroni will have damaged many parts of my abdominal compartment and gastrointestinal tract as it passed from my oesophagus at the top, into my stomach, to the small intestines and eventually out from my large intestines after being metabolised by my liver.

Rather than the ethanol itself in your craft beer, mojito or negroni, it is the metabolism of the ethanol by your liver cells into the poisonous yet fruity-smelling chemicals – acetaldehyde and acetate – that changes the brain and causes you to dance the way you did at last year's Christmas party. These products have a predilection for the frontal lobes of the brain, responsible for behaviour, and for the body's balance centre, the cerebellum. They reduce our inhibitions, promote hunger, increase aggression and unleash sexual disinhibition. Similarly, these chemical breakdown products then move on to inflict harm on the cells in our liver, day after day, little by little.

It is often said that drinking alcohol is like borrowing happiness from tomorrow. Many of us associate drinking alcohol with celebrations, holidays, a fine meal and fun times. For others, as George Bernard Shaw is supposed to have said, 'alcohol is the anaesthesia by which we endure the operation of life'. The reasons we drink alcohol may vary from person to person, but the physical effects will be the same.

~

My long runs of shifts spent at the hospital sometimes feel like being far away at sea: I speak to the same people, eat the same food and inhale the same smells for days at a time. I could understand why Louie would regularly drink alcohol in his downtime at sea during his twenty years serving in the merchant navy. Although the whisky didn't alter the material facts surrounding him, it did change his perception of those facts. It took off the salty hard edge.

Now in his seventies, having travelled the seas to every continent except Antarctica, Louie worried that the past was catching up with him. His trousers no longer fitted over his swollen abdomen. The whites of his eyes were not white. He didn't sleep well. Five days before his seventy-first birthday, Louie vomited blood – a great deal of blood. I know because my new shoes were covered with it after the team had put Louie onto a life-support machine. It was my first week as a junior doctor.

The liver is an amazing beast of an organ, weighing over 1.5 kg. It receives a quarter of all the blood pumped out from your heart every minute. It is so beautifully complex yet looks so unassuming, hiding more than 500 functions beneath a sheen of purple-pink. Unlike other organs, despite decades of trying, it is still not possible to replicate its functions using machines. Thankfully, like a character from a superhero comic, the liver has the incredible ability to regrow. It needs just a quarter of its original tissue to help spawn new liver cells. Its roles go far beyond that of the 'detoxification' that sustains so-called health-food retailers' post-Christmas marketing campaigns. Hormone production, blood clotting, drug metabolism, temperature regulation, fat synthesis, digestion and even our sex drive are in part controlled by this organ. It is the open-plan kitchen of your body, where most activities occur at some point.

It is no wonder, then, that Louie's liver disease had led so easily to his critical illness. While, globally, infections of the liver are the most common reasons for its failure, it is unsurprising that alcohol consumption is the leading cause in the Western world. In over one-third of patients with liver failure, alcohol is the prime cause and one in two liver transplants occur as a result of liver failure from alcohol misuse. It may shock you to learn that overall alcoholic liver disease has been estimated to kill more people than diabetes and road collisions combined.

Once Louie was stabilised in intensive care, we had time to think. Listening to his story and examining his body, we already had a good indication of what had happened. Louie's alcohol consumption had been excessive for years. Those breakdown products that allowed Louie to become detached from his salt-crusted reality had been inflicting minor degrees of liver damage with every drink. While alcohol can occasionally cause a rapid, dramatic inflammation of the liver called alcoholic hepatitis, more commonly it inflicts silent, repeated damage. The scarring that resulted turned Louie's liver from a pink, soft, forgiving workhorse into a big, hard, bobbled, yellow problem. Liver cirrhosis ensued, borrowing the Greek word 'kirrhos' to describe the resulting yellow, tawny appearance to the damaged organ.

We knew Louie had liver cirrhosis after curling our fingers underneath his ribcage on the right-hand side of his body. His enlarged liver pressed against my hand, making its presence known. Press down now with the flats of your left-hand fingers, just under your ribcage on the right, and take a deep breath in. You may feel a gentle nudge from your healthy liver on the top side of your index finger. If you had done this on Louie's abdomen, you would feel his liver reaching across to his umbilicus, or belly button.

As it gradually failed, Louie's liver also stopped breaking down oestrogen hormones normally found in small amounts in men. Multiple spider-shaped blood vessels started sprouting over his chest, just like in women during pregnancy, and increased levels of female hormones then caused growth of residual breast tissue.

By using our hands and our heads we were able to make sense of Louie's story. Then his blood tests and liver scan confirmed our fears: his blood-clotting system had also failed, as his liver had stopped making the proteins that normally stop a cut from bleeding. But this wasn't enough to explain why he was vomiting so much blood. For this we needed to use our eyes as well as our hands and heads. We needed to look inside Louie's gut – from his mouth, down his food pipe into his stomach and out into his small intestine. The blood that had landed on my shoes must have come from somewhere along this route, so a metre-long flexible endoscope, the width of your index finger, was inserted into his mouth. Sometimes called the 'magic eye', the endoscope exploits fibre-optic technology of the 1950s to allow us to literally see inside the human body. Today, thanks to miniaturised LED cameras used in place of direct optics, endoscopes are the first step in investigating gastro-intestinal bleeding.

The tiny camera deep inside Louie's body flashed up live images on the adjacent television screen just like a breaking news report. The moment we entered his oesophagus, the source of bleeding was obvious. The normally smooth side walls of his food pipe had been replaced by thick, engorged, pulsating blood vessels, like snakes climbing its walls. These oesophageal varices were veins desperately trying to find a way of returning blood to the heart after their normal route through the liver had become blocked by scar tissue. It was the body's way of bypassing roadworks in Louie's liver, only this time the main route was closed for good. The diversion that these veins took was a route not used to such high volumes of bloody traffic. The vessel walls were thin and made of weak materials and so Louie's side roads had burst under the strain.

The endoscope used to see those varices had a thin chan-nel through which devices could be passed. The bleeding was soon shut down by strong stainless-steel clips that were pushed down the endoscope before being clasped around Louie's bulging veins. Suddenly, one flew off under the sheer pressure, forcing spurts of blood to cover the camera lens, projected onto the large screen transmitting the images from inside Louie's body. We stepped back in surprise as the scope was quickly withdrawn, the camera at the tip wiped before being plunged back into Louie's mouth. A fresh clip was quickly secured to the bleeding vein before the scene was transformed into a sea of red.

Oesophageal varices are just one of the life-threatening consequences of liver cirrhosis. Expanded blood vessels can occur in other places that have large networks of veins, including the rectum, vagina and the abdominal wall where they are called *caput medusa* after their resemblance to the snakes of the Greek Gorgon's hair. Cirrhosis also markedly increases the chances of developing liver cancer. In addition, Louie's trousers no longer fitted due to another complication in which venous back pressure from a blocked, scarred liver causes up to 20 litres of fluid to accumulate within the abdomen. Microbes find this fluid pleasant as a growth medium, after creeping across the bowel wall, infecting the abdominal spaces. Any one of these problems can tip the balance towards full liver failure.

Although we managed to stop Louie's bleeding using the endoscope, his liver was still struggling. The yellow of his once-white eyes indicated that the bile salts normally broken down by the liver were building up. No sedative drugs had been given for days, yet he still remained deeply unconscious from the toxins no longer removed by his damaged liver. Measuring the level of ammonia in Louie's blood, we confirmed that his liver had stopped filtering waste substances that can put the brain to sleep. Even more worrying were the recurrent small bleeds we found when removing fluid from his stomach using a tube inserted through his nose: in spite of the clipping procedure, his oesophageal varices were still causing problems.

The only remaining solution was to make a new connection between the blood vessels leading into and out of his liver. We considered building a flyover (a shunt) to allow blood to drive around the congested roads inside his liver, but this procedure reduces even further the filtering of waste materials and so patients will often become increasingly confused and sedated as a result. Therefore, we persevered with supportive treatments in intensive care and waited until Louie started to wake up three days later. Although his liver failure was still present, it had stopped getting worse. After we were able to take Louie off the life-support machine, he would later tell the nurses that he thought he had been at sea. He was thin, weak and malnourished despite being fed through a tube and the poor man looked more like he had been shipwrecked.

Even with extra protein being added to his feeding regime, Louie became a shadow of his former self after only five days of illness and needed twice-daily physiotherapy, even when unconscious, simply to retain any of the muscles he would need if he was ever to walk again. We are used to this daily struggle to maintain muscle strength and we have teams of specially trained physiotherapists who form a cornerstone of supportive rehabilitation in intensive care. Why, then, even after providing adequate calories, would Louie become so thin and weak so quickly?

Critical illness dramatically changes the way your body

deals with nutrition. Despite an excess of calories delivered to patients in intensive care via feeding tubes, they will lose as much as 20 per cent of their muscle mass within three days. High levels of stress hormones contribute towards this body-reshaping, as anyone with anxiety will know. The mechanical work performed by our breathing machines also thins the diaphragm after just twenty-four hours of use. Genes controlling muscle strength switch off after only two hours of using this equipment. Unlike much of society, Louie's challenge now was to put on weight rather than to lose it.

The story of humanity could cynically be summarised as a 200,000-year-long struggle for food, water and sex. Everything after that – conflict, power, corruption, love, society or even medicine – was a descendant of these first needs. Today, more people die from overnutrition than undernutrition. If ethanol is the most destructive substance in Western society, carbohydrates come a close second. The obesity epidemic is rapidly growing irrespective of copious well-meaning education. We need to change our equipment in hospitals to simply cope with this new challenge: stronger and bigger beds, and hoists. We need specialist staff training on how to lift heavy weights and have even increased the width of doorways. Occasionally body scanners designed for zoo animals have been considered to help get a diagnosis in humans. It is quickly becoming apparent that the last fifty years' accepted wisdom of promoting a low-fat diet has backfired in a spectacular sense. The finger now points towards refined carbohydrates found – and often cleverly hidden – in cakes, white bread and sugary drinks as the main culprit in weight gain and ill health. The misleading campaigns offering 'low-fat' alternatives may have conversely led to escalating levels of obesity due to replacement of fat content with refined sugars. Sadly, our hard-wired, insatiable appetite for sweet treats is tough to shake off due to their dense calorific content, essential for survival in the past. The selfish gene's most successful ploy – the love of food – may be humanity's biggest challenge.

Visiting Louie on the liver ward a few days after he had been discharged from intensive care, I looked at his blood tests and was concerned to see that he was once again developing liver failure. His medical notes explained that he was still vomiting blood and yet the bypass procedure we had considered before had still not been done. I was confused: why were we not doing the only thing that could help?

After I spoke to Louie, the answer became clear. I had fallen into the common trap of being focused only on what is possible rather than what is preferable. Louie was frail and his health had been deteriorating over the last ten months rather than simply the last ten days since I had first met him. Louie described to me with great lucidity and passion what 'a life worth living' meant to him. He had been clinging onto independence, but even leaving the house over the last few months had been a real struggle. Louie wanted us to offer treatments that would give him back the independent life that he knew and loved. Going back to the intensive care unit for a second time with multi-organ failure would not do this. Nothing would. And he knew this, so what Louie really wanted now was simple: he asked me for a drink, not of alcohol, but of water.

I considered carefully whether I should give Louie a drink of water. He still had a tube in his nose, draining small amounts of blood. He was coughing – what if he choked? Was it safe? Reading through his notes, the medical team had come to the same conclusion as Louie: further aggressive medical treatment would no longer be in his best interests. It was unlikely to work, and, even if it did, Louie would never have his independence back due to the severity of his illness and chronic health conditions. Instead, we focused our energy on relieving symptoms rather than striving for a cure. Louie was thirsty, and I could help with that.

I poured Louie a glass of water, and lifted it to his dry, cracked lips. As his Adam's apple moved in time with his swallow, he opened his eyes, looked at me and then smiled. His gravelly voice said: 'Thanks, boy. That's like coins falling from heaven.' This simple act of giving a drink was one of the most satisfying experiences during my first year as a junior doctor. I later went to say goodbye to Louie after my shift had ended. As I turned away to leave the ward, Louie leant forwards as a huge wave of fresh blood hurtled onto the floor with a splash. Minutes later, he died.

That night I went out for food with my family. I thought about Louie a lot. I drank my customary cold beer as I ate my meal. Was I wrong to do this? How could I separate what I had seen only hours earlier from what I was doing now? Sometimes I feel like a hypocrite when I don't always follow my own advice. The balance between 'you only live once' and living well is a delicate one, and I certainly don't have any easy answers.

~

Dani was just twenty-one years old when she was diagnosed with Crohn's disease. Named after New York physician Dr Burrill Crohn in 1932, this is an immune disorder affecting the entire gastrointestinal tract anywhere between your lips and your anus. Dr Crohn researched the disease until he retired at the age of ninety. He discovered that, rather than the immune system behaving as a surveillance mechanism, responding only to harmful pathogens, it can turn against itself, attacking the delicate lining of the bowel. Like many autoimmune diseases, the exact cause of this change from helper to hunter is unclear, but likely reasons include environmental infections, genetic predisposition and lifestyle choices. In the short term, these attacks produce diarrhoea, discomfort and weight loss. Today, with steroids, modern immune drugs and patient education, the disease can be successfully managed by most people without anyone other than their close friends and family being aware of their battles. However, in some people with frequent, recurrent and severe bouts of the disease, it can be deadly.

Like any injured tissue, the bowel tries to repair itself after these attacks. If the insult arrives frequently and tirelessly, the resulting repair mechanisms produce scarring. Unlike a scar on your face, scarring of your bowel has more profound consequences than simply a cosmetic challenge: this scar tissue can swell, split and stick together. When the hollow tubes of the bowels connect together they can form channels called fistulae, resulting in their contents leaking from one into another. Scarring can also produce blockages, with the resulting back pressure causing spasms of pain as the bowel tries to contract. Dani had suffered from all of these complications.

Ten years before we met Dani she had a severe flare-up of her Crohn's disease, despite her condition being treated with powerful immune-modulating drugs. The days it normally took for symptoms to pass turned into weeks. One morning, the pain in her abdomen had been so severe that she went into hospital. When Dani came out, she would never eat normally again.

The pain she experienced in that flare-up was down to an 'acute abdomen'. When a surgeon pressed down on her stomach, the pain would sharply increase and the muscles of her abdominal wall became as rigid as a board. These are the signs that the thin protective lining of her abdomen, the peritoneum, was inflamed due to a catastrophe inside. Her muscles were contracting to guard her vital organs. The causes of an acute abdomen are far- and wide-reaching. Most commonly, it can result from a bowel inflammation or a perforation. This may occur due to appendicitis or diverticular disease, where small sacs in the bowel wall, formed after years of constipation, become infected. Other causes include stomach ulcers that rupture, blood vessels that burst, lack of blood supply to the bowel or infections of the gallbladder and liver.

Dani had had a scan on her abdomen that told a very difficult surgical story: multiple loops of her 5-metre-long small bowel were stuck together, with false connections between these loops and areas of complete blockage. There was also evidence of severe infection where her bowel contents were leaking through holes in the intestine wall. Dani needed a major operation called a laparotomy. A surgeon would first cut through her skin, then through the muscle and connective-tissue layers in the middle of her abdomen to reveal the organs inside. Just getting to this stage is difficult and dangerous even before any repairs can be started.

A laparotomy is the most common operation to result in critical illness. Even where the underlying gut problem is relatively minor, the procedure needed to access the abdominal organs can leave patients fighting to survive. Sometimes it is possible to use keyhole techniques, where plastic tubes are inserted through multiple 1 cm openings to allow cameras to look internally and direct instruments to fix any problems. The abdominal cavity is inflated with up to 50 litres of gas every hour, causing it to bulge upwards like a domed tent glowing red from the camera lights inside. Early trials of this technique using oxygen as the gas blown in were less than successful, literally leading to fires in the belly. There are few worse places for a fire. Now that oxygen has been replaced by a gas used in fire extinguishers (carbon dioxide), this is thankfully impossible. Using carbon dioxide means it is safe to use electricity to gently burn the edges of dissected tissue, which helps to reduce bleeding.

While there have been significant advances in laparoscopic (keyhole) surgery, including robotic assistance, there are times when using this keyhole technique is simply not possible. The complexity of Dani's bowel anatomy – with its multiple connections, holes and blockages – was too great to be operated upon using cameras alone. It needed the most advanced surgical technology we still have today: the human eyeball and the opposable thumb of the surgical human hand.

Laparotomies result in three main challenges for patients. Firstly, opening the abdominal contents to the cold air outside and handling them causes great fluid shifts and losses. Your body consists of 75 per cent water. While reading this page, you are losing around 70 ml of fluid per hour through breathing, urine production and sweat. If you are reading this while on holiday, lying next to the pool or at the beach, you may lose double this amount. If I were to cut into your abdomen and simply do nothing, you would lose over 400 ml of fluid per hour through evaporation alone – even before any blood loss from my surgical technique. When you become critically ill, the delicate lining of blood vessels and organs breaks down and allows fluid to seep out. Simply matching any fluid losses will cause swelling of the face, arms and even the bowels themselves. We therefore replace these losses using intravenous fluids and monitors to carefully guide how much to give.

The second challenge after a laparotomy is infection. Whenever a compartment of the body is opened, bugs move in. This is true even in the seemingly sterile environment of an operating theatre. Sterility is never truly achieved, as even killing 99.9 per cent of microbes leaves millions behind. Some diseases, such as bowel perforation, result in the contents of the bowels being spilt into the abdominal compartment, resulting in severe infection. These are often polymicrobial infections, with a mixture of different organisms normally found in faeces, including fungal species.

The final challenge facing patients recovering after surgery is the most significant and is the reason why, ten years ago, Dani became critically ill after her laparotomy. The mechanics of human breathing rely upon stable abdominal musculature, a powerful diaphragm moving freely and the ability to cough. All of these mechanisms are impaired once the abdominal wall has been divided for a laparotomy: the muscles are split, the diaphragm splinted due to pain, and coughing can be difficult. We try to reduce the likelihood of these complications by employing pain-relief strategies including epidurals and pain pumps, but there are risks and benefits to all of these interventions. Dani's severe infection at the time of her surgery meant that the risks of inserting an epidural into her spine were too high, which in turn meant that breathing was difficult, painful and ineffective after her ten-hour operation. She would spend three days on a breathing machine to give her body time to recover.

Due to the complexity of Dani's disease, simply fixing the blockages and abnormal connections in her bowel had not been possible. Instead the surgeon had needed to physically remove most of her intestine. Out of the original 5 metres, she was left with just 20 cm of bowel. This was not enough. The intestine not only extracts fluid and energy from our diet, but it also plays a key role in absorbing vitamins and minerals. With just 20 cm of bowel, Dani was no longer able to absorb sufficient calories, nutrients, fluid or vitamins. Thirty years ago, Dani would have gradually withered away and died. Fortunately, when she became critically ill ten years before I met her, there was something that could be done: her life was saved thanks to food being injected directly into her bloodstream.

Total parenteral nutrition (TPN) was first used in 1969 by doctors treating newborns with bowel cancer. It is a fluid containing all the essential elements of a nutritionally balanced diet in their most basic form, which is injected directly into the blood rather than absorbed through the bowel. In Dani's case, her bowel was not long enough to absorb even the most basic nutrients needed for life and so an alternative route was needed. Rather than delivering Dani's nutrition through her gastrointestinal system, it would be directly inserted into her bloodstream.

TPN, with its high fat and salt content, cannot simply be injected through the veins of the hand. Instead, it needs to be infused through large central veins. Its sugars, proteins and fats also offer a perfect medium to grow microorganisms and so, exploiting the protective system of the skin, we tunnel specialised plastic lines under portions of the body surface before they dive deep down into blood vessels. The plastic tunnels are left permanently in the body, allowing liquid food to be infused by patients at home. Along with careful handling of the open ends of these lines, this minimises the chances of infections in these foreign materials.

I met Dani a decade after she had eaten her first meal using her bloodstream rather than her mouth. While I had lost count of the number of restaurants I had visited in that time, Dani had not: zero is an easy number to remember. Although she could taste flavours in small quantities, she had not eaten a meal in ten years. This strikes me as both amazing and terrible at the same time. As medicine solves one problem, it creates others.

While a patient was complaining about the quality of the hospital food, Dani told me she would give anything to simply experience eating that terrible meal. Food, buying, preparing and eating it, is at the centre of many of our daily experiences. I might nibble on olives at a party, buy overpriced popcorn at the cinema and taste the birthday cake of my nine-year-old daughter. None of these are directly aimed at providing nutrition. Rather, they enrich the human experience – something that TPN could never do. However, as a strong, independent and inspirational woman, Dani didn't let this stop her. With tenacity and courage, she would join friends at those restaurants and parties, having a variety of chewing gums to match the mood and the course being served. She carried her food pump in an expensive designer bag and wasn't embarrassed to show her scars during the rare hot British summer.

When I met her, a severe infection had brought Dani back to the same ICU where she had recovered ten years previously. We were worried that another abdominal catastrophe had occurred, made worse by the immune drugs she was still taking to keep her Crohn's disease in remission. Thankfully her abdominal scans were reassuring. We turned our focus instead towards the foreign plastic that had been inside her body for longer than my daughter had been alive. We took the difficult but essential step of removing her tunnelled line as a potential source of infection. We were not 100 per cent sure if we were right, but happily the decision we took to remove this lifeline was the correct one. The plastic tube that had been keeping her alive had, in fact, nearly killed her by growing bacteria and fungi that had been thriving on the food she needed to live. After her second period of three days in intensive care, Dani was back to her normal self. Before she went home, a new tunnel line was inserted and soon the food pump could be placed back inside her leather handbag.

In the ICU we will continue to meet patients with gut problems. Through our doors will come patients following major surgery from cancer and infections, and we will encounter patients with stomach ulcers that have ruptured and food pipes that have burst from profuse vomiting. Bowel cancer will lead to critical illness when a hidden tumour leaks and when the operation needed to remove the cancer is difficult and long. And we will be ready to fight for the survival of these patients.

Today, your chances of surviving after a laparotomy are double those of forty years ago. We have new surgical instruments that can join bowels back together more quickly and safely than ever before. We have learnt lessons from space exploration on how to nourish and maintain the body's muscles when under extreme stress. Machines that replace the functions of the liver and pancreas are already in medical trials, which will give patients the time they need to survive. So long as patients have fires in their belly, there will be intensive care professionals ready to put them out.

8

THE BLOOD

The emulsion of life

Carl Sagan, one of the most celebrated scientists of the last 100 years, famously said, 'We are made of star-stuff.' In a violent process deep inside a giant red star billions of years ago, the light atoms of helium, carbon and oxygen were crushed together, forming the heaviest atom type a star can muster. At that moment, the star transformed into a supernova, exploding and showering the universe with iron. Now 4 grams of that 'star-stuff' is inside the veins in your hands as they hold this book. This iron is what gives our blood its deep-red stain, and allows mammals to breathe oxygen-rich air and remove waste carbon dioxide from our metabolic processes. It was also the first metal forged by our ancestors into weapons to spill the blood of others.

Iron is a key component of the haemoglobin molecule, packaged inside the 30 trillion red blood cells that speed around your body at 5 litres per minute. Haemoglobin allows oxygen to bind to its surface, moving it from the lungs to every cell in your body. It simultaneously allows carbon dioxide produced by aerobic metabolism to be transported back to the lungs and removed as we breathe out. Along with red cells, our blood is an emulsion of white blood cells, platelets, proteins and water. If you drained all of the blood from your body, it would soon fill around seven wine bottles.

If you tried to prove this fact, though, you would not be able to pour it back in because evolution has produced an extremely efficient system of blood-clotting. A near-instantaneous reaction occurs between blood cells and proteins as soon as tissue is damaged. The cascading reaction snowballs, calling additional cells to action while laying down temporary scaffolding, blocking any escape routes and even causing blood vessels to contract. Your body will do all it can to prevent the escape of blood and preserve your life.

Throughout the often-aggressive 6 million years of human evolution, this response has been a helpful one. It has allowed us to survive falls, animal attacks and human attacks. But those same survival adaptions now endanger the lives of sedentary, sofa-lying humans. Today's inactive, desk-sitting life stops blood from being moved around. Lack of regular muscle contractions leads to stationary blood, which leads to sticky blood, which leads to blood clots. The balance between your blood clotting too easily or not at all is an adjustable fine line. If I were to use ultrasound waves to scan your calf veins, I would be twice as likely to discover a blood clot after a long-haul flight. This demonstrates that even a short period of immobility – combined with minor dehydration and low oxygen tension from pressurised aircraft cabins – is sufficient to impact your clotting system. Imagine, then, the factors implicit during critical illness and it will be little surprise that blood clots are common in intensive care patients. The incidence of these minor blood clots nears 30 per cent in the critically ill, who are forced to be sedentary because of their condition. These small clots are often the consequence of being ill rather than the cause and so require no treatment, yet developing a new major blood clot can kill.

One name associated with this area of medicine is that of Rudolf Ludwig Carl Virchow, a German physician during the nineteenth century who would have struggled to fit into today's structured medical training programme. He was an anthropologist, pathologist, prehistorian, biologist, writer, editor, politician and public health visionary. It is no wonder that his friends described him as the 'pope of medicine'. He described how blood clots are able to form in the veins of the leg before travelling through the chambers of the heart to become lodged in the arteries that supply the lungs. We call these blood clots pulmonary emboli and, as a result of his hard work, we call the three factors – injury to blood vessels, increased blood stickiness and low flow rates – that lead to their development 'Virchow's triad'.

The most severely ill patients spend days lying on their

backs, not even moving their eyelids, and so intensive care patients invariably fulfil all of Virchow's factors. They will have fluid pushed into and pulled out of their bodies through bleeding, transfusions and treatments, and their blood vessels will be injured by needles and foreign plastic pipes being slid in and out. Furthermore, the very diseases that they are suffering from may additionally predispose them to blood clots.

There are few evidence-based treatments that have been shown definitively to cure disease in critical care – in my opinion, these are restricted to antibiotics, steroids, surgery and time – and so a key goal of intensive care medicine should be to avoid future harm while supporting the organs and providing these limited, effective treatments in good measure. A blood clot is one common complication of critical illness we aim to prevent by using both physical devices to promote blood flow in the legs and drugs to reduce the coagulability of the blood. Even with all of these efforts, nearly one-third of critically ill patients will develop blood clots.

～

Melody was raised by her mum following her dad's death when she was just five years old, and she flitted through life like a firefly in a candlelit vigil. Expelled from school, and later sacked from more jobs than she had fingers to count, her only constants were drugs and homelessness. Her road to ill health was a well-trodden one, starting with alcohol, then progressing to cannabis before Melody tore the first hole in her veins to inject drugs at the age of nineteen.

We met Melody in the small hours of the morning on a windy, rainy Saturday. A homeless-charity worker had brought her to the emergency department, rightly worried about her breathing. Melody showed all the cardinal features of pneumonia. The severity of her illness necessitated her being swiftly placed onto a life-support machine. Over the next two days in intensive care, Melody gradually improved, with decreasing amounts of oxygen needed and her blood pressure no longer having to be supported by powerful drugs. Then, without warning, at 7 a.m. on the third day, her heart stopped.

My colleague Dr Holmes arrived at Melody's bedside just in time. The team had already been doing CPR for a few minutes without success. Quickly recapping the story aloud, Dr Holmes' brain fired a warning shot. This was a young woman who had been getting better not worse. She had had a sudden deterioration that resulted in a cardiac arrest. In the few minutes prior to this, she had suddenly needed more oxygen. This didn't fit with a heart problem or even with a worsening of her infection. This sounded like a big blood clot had gone to her lungs, although there was no time to confirm this with a full CT scan. Blindly giving the clot-busting and blood-thinning treatments for a pulmonary embolus could result in severe bleeding all over the body, especially into Melody's brain. Dr Holmes needed more evidence before taking these risks, but every second he waited Melody's brain struggled with no oxygen. To get an answer, he reached for a machine waiting silently in the corner: he used ultrasound on Melody's heart.

Although you may not have realised, you probably used ultrasound today. Did you charge your toothbrush or phone without needing to plug it in? Were you helped to park your car using a parking sensor? Perhaps you heard a burglar alarm when its soundwaves were disturbed by an intruder? Human hearing can distinguish sounds of frequencies up to 20 kHz. Above this level, sounds are undetectable by our auditory system – they are ultra (beyond) sound. If this were not the case, you would hear the constant gnawing of signals pulsing through wires, of everyday objects vibrating, and animals communicating. Just like your car radio, the higher the frequency of these waves, the better the quality of the signal received. This is why listening to music using short-wave FM radio is a better experience than tuning in to a long-wave station. The longer the wavelength, the lower the frequency, the worse the quality. These longer wavelengths do have some advantages. The last time you drove through a tunnel or around a mountain range, the short-wave FM radio will have quickly faded while the foreign-language long-wave radio stations remained. These lower-frequency sound waves may not have a good acoustic quality but they can penetrate very effectively.

Producing medical images using ultrasound was first introduced in 1942 by Austrian Dr Karl Theodore Dussik, who used it to diagnose tumours of the brain. He turned vibrations made by sound waves moving through tissue into images that look like slices through the body. The practical applications were significantly improved by the Scottish professor Ian Donald in the 1950s after he saw it being used in the shipyards of Glasgow to identify flaws in metal seams. After becoming Professor of Midwifery at the University of Glasgow, he used these 'metal flaw detector' techniques to instead find human flaws. Today we can look at the unborn faces of our children in the womb thanks to his invention. The development of obstetric ultrasound is probably still the best-known use of this technology today, but if you have ever had a scan of your heart, your gallbladder, your liver, your aorta or even your kidneys it was probably thanks to ultrasound.

With the advent of modern, portable, high-quality, affordable machines, ultrasound has transformed the practice of intensive care medicine. Although first used by doctors to insert needles safely into blood vessels, I now use ultrasound on patients every day. I look at the structures in their neck, the valves of their heart, the lining of their lungs, the size of their kidneys, blood vessels in their liver and arms, and even the nerves at the back of their eyes. Structures close to the body surface can be viewed in beautiful, high-quality images by using high-frequency probes of up to 10 MHz. You can distinguish tendons, blood vessels and nerves in your arm simply by their appearance on a screen. Deeper areas, such as the kidneys, need slower, longer waves at around 3 MHz to penetrate your muscle and fat. All of this can be done at the bedside or even at the side of the road following a car accident. Ultrasound is part of a rapid yet accurate assessment of what has caused a patient to become critically unwell and it can direct the right treatment to the right patient at the right time.

When Dr Holmes' brain fired that warning shot about Melody's sudden cardiac arrest, he was able to call on his additional training with ultrasound to image the heart to a level normally performed by heart specialists. Using a cardiac ultrasound probe, he quickly looked at Melody's barely beating heart. At once he could see a hugely enlarged right ventricle that normally pumps blood to the lungs. The presence of any blockage between the right side of the heart and the lungs causes back pressure leading to such an enlargement. Armed with this evidence, combined with his cognitive insight, he was able to make a difficult call: he injected a high dose of a clot-busting drug that would smash apart any blood clots throughout Melody's body. The drug was indiscriminate, which left Melody at risk of severe bleeding. Although we would see any bleeding on the outside of her body, it was impossible to tell if there was bleeding inside. As the team continued to do CPR, pressing hard up and down on Melody's chest, the image on the ultrasound screen slowly started to change. Melody's weakly squeezing heart motion became gradually stronger and stronger until, twenty minutes later, it was beating soundly all by itself. Her oxygen levels increased, her kidneys started to produce urine and her brain appeared to be intact as her pupils reacted to light.

When I met Melody later that morning, she was stable enough to have a scan of her lungs and brain. Dr Holmes sent me a message that afternoon as he struggled to sleep after his eventful night shift, and I was delighted to tell him that he had made the right call. Melody's lung scan had shown a massive blood clot straddling the division between the main arteries supplying her lungs with blood, and her brain scan had shown no bleeding. Dr Holmes had used the right treatment in the right patient at the right time, and five days later Melody self-discharged from the intensive care unit.

~

During my early years as a junior doctor, I worked with an inspirational surgeon called Mr Ruddle. His specialism of vascular surgery aims to repair the blood vessels that carry our iron-stained emulsion of life. One poor decision or surgical slip can end with a lot of spilt blood. Mr Ruddle was a great surgeon, knowing not only how and when to operate, but also when not to operate. His life outside of medicine was as fascinating as watching him operate. While I would spend my annual leave camping in Cornwall or seeking respite from the Welsh winter in sunnier climes, he would ride bareback horses across the mountains of Afghanistan, surf Hawaii's big wave known as 'Jaws' or climb Mount Everest. During the arrival of a yellowing autumn after returning from another adventure, his surf van would be put to a very different use: this time to save a life.

As Tristan sat down in the early autumn light after a sleepless night, he couldn't know that an hour later he would be critically ill. The painkiller he had taken last night had done little for the pain in his abdomen. It seemed to continuously tear through his centre into the muscles of his back. But Tristan's decades of working in the clanging heart of Wales' industrial furnace-roaring steel industry had made him a tough man. He seldom complained, and he never saw his doctor. Except for this week. He made sure that he sat close to the telephone in case the results of his scan from a few days ago were available. Sure enough, at 8 a.m. the old-fashioned telephone bell rang out, but it wasn't the voice of his general practitioner he had been expecting on the line.

Mr Ruddle had woken at the same time as Tristan, having just returned from a trip to India. He turned the key in his VW surf van and drove to work early, ready for his non-clinical day catching up on paperwork. Underneath his office door had been slipped a scan result with 'URGENT' written in red pen along the front. The scan report did not make good reading. Before his eyes had reached the end of the final sentence, Mr Ruddle picked up his office phone and dialled an unfamiliar number. Tristan answered. He was still alive – that was a good start.

The largest blood vessel in the body is the abdominal aorta. Normally just 2 cm in diameter, it originates from the left side of the heart. Its first branches are to the coronary arteries, which supply the heart with its own blood. It then curves around into the shape of a horseshoe, with its next divisions going to the head and chest. Finally, it descends between the lungs then squeezes through an opening in the diaphragm, at which point it becomes the abdominal aorta.

The stress placed on the abdominal aorta, even when we are healthy, is high. If this is compounded by high blood pressure, breakdown of vessel elasticity from smoking or high cholesterol, these mechanical stresses can become too much for it. Should the integrity of the vessel wall become compromised due to a tear, blood will soon escape. Initially, small volumes of blood may tear at the aorta's layers, stripping them apart from the inside and creating a 'false' channel through which further blood can escape. If this happens at the front of the vessel, blood breaks into the open abdominal cavity and the outcome is rapid death from catastrophic blood loss. The back of the abdominal aorta, however, lies behind the abdominal cavity, surrounded by strong layers of connective tissues and muscles called the retroperitoneal space. This allows a 'tamponade' of any bleeding where the pressure outside of an open hole equalises to that inside, thereby temporarily stopping blood flow. How long this false stability lasts is difficult to predict – sometimes it will be minutes, sometimes hours, rarely days. What will occur is severe abdominal pain that tears through into the back. Exactly like Tristan had.

Just minutes after Tristan's phone rang there came a knock at his door. Through his window, he could see an unfamiliar grey van with its engine still running. As Tristan opened the front door, Mr Ruddle said: 'Hi, Tristan. Sorry to come so quickly, but I really need to get you to the hospital.'

Reading Tristan's scan report, Mr Ruddle knew that he had little time to waste. Tristan had an enormous 7 cm abdominal aortic aneurysm that had ruptured into his retroperitoneal space, and without an operation he would die. Tristan lived just minutes from the hospital so, rather than delay for an ambulance, Mr Ruddle drove to Tristan's house, lifted him cautiously onto the bed in the back of his surf van and drove carefully to the hospital. He had already told the emergency operating theatre so they could prepare for what was needed next. He called the ICU, knowing that Tristan would need all of their machines and care if he even survived the operation. He then rang the on-call anaesthetist. During that period of my training, that person was me.

The methods used to repair blood vessels were brought to the forefront by the Lebanese-American surgeon, Dr Michael DeBakey. His life was nothing short of special. He discovered early links between smoking and lung cancer, performed one of the world's first heart-bypass surgeries and introduced operations still essential to save lives in my hospital today. He even trialled the first mechanical heart device that is now fast becoming a reasonable alternative to a heart transplant for some patients. Dr DeBakey continued working until the age of ninety-nine after suffering a catastrophic aneurysm rupture himself aged ninety-seven.

His life was saved by a seven-hour operation that he had invented, followed by a prolonged stay in the ICU. He died two months before his 100th birthday.

Like many major operations, the success of the 'anatomical' repair is only the starting point for patient survival. The physiological stress that a major operation places on a patient is similar to them being in a major road traffic accident: it increases the need for oxygen by all the major organ systems, it demands more from the heart, and the kidneys react by retaining water and reducing blood flow. Major operations increase the risks of heart attacks, strokes, infections, kidney failure and liver failure. Therefore – as with all areas of medicine – the surgeon, the stitch and the operation are only parts of the orchestra needed to play together in unison to promote life.

As I used anaesthetic drugs best suited to Tristan's disease, his eyes slowly closed. We needed to maintain his blood pressure to ensure adequate flow to his organs yet prevent it being too high and leading to further bleeding. Using painkillers a hundred times more powerful than heroin, we prevented Tristan's body from reacting as a breathing tube was inserted into his trachea. We monitored his brainwaves, using just the right amount of anaesthetic for unconsciousness while minimising its effect on the rest of his body. Short, plastic tubes with a large diameter were inserted into his veins, exploiting theories of fluid dynamics to increase flow rates as blood was transfused. All of this was done in the middle of an operating theatre, with Mr Ruddle holding a knife in his right hand. The anaesthetic would relax the muscles around the retroperitoneal space, thereby removing the only force preventing Tristan from bleeding to death, and so Mr Ruddle needed to be ready to operate within seconds of the anaesthetic agents taking effect.

It was clear within minutes of starting the operation that Tristan's life was hanging by a thread. Gushes of blood were being suctioned into the plastic tubes designed to clear the operating field as quickly as we could push new blood back into Tristan. This leaking blood was not wasted: a cell-saver machine used centrifugal forces to separate out the red blood cells before we transfused them back into Tristan's body. As blood exited the hole in his aorta, the machine forced it under pressure back through more plastic tubes into his veins.

Tristan's temperature had to be kept normal so that his blood clotted correctly. We warmed extra donated blood using machines that circulated heated water around the pipes carrying the blood – just like an underfloor heating system. However, while we can do much using drugs and equipment to reduce bleeding, when there is a big leak, it simply needs to be stopped. Tristan's main problem was not that he was cold, or his clotting system was broken, or that he lacked clotting drugs. His problem was that there was a large hole in his aorta – in essence, the tap needed to be turned off. Mr Ruddle called for assistance from his surgical colleagues but, in the meantime, there was only one thing I could do to help. I was standing on one side of the patient's drapes with a senior consultant anaesthetist, looking at Tristan's vital signs and using powerful drugs, but I was more needed on the other side.

Medicine, like other industries, is heavily invested in tribalism. This can improve team cohesion and it can allow trust to be built up quickly between relative strangers, but it can also destroy good patient care. One day you may work with a surgical team, criticising how non-surgical teams manage patients. The next day, you change sides, turning your frustration or anger towards your old tribe. In emergencies such as Tristan's, there is no time for tribalism. Although my tribe at that time was the anaesthetic team, Tristan needed me to be something else. He needed his bleeding to be stopped by the surgeon, and I was a pair of hands that could help. I stepped the other side of the drapes separating surgeon from anaesthetist and soon, wearing a surgical gown, I too had my hands inside of Tristan. The job I did required little skill – I simply held back Tristan's tissues and removed blood using a sucker – but this simple act allowed Mr Ruddle to see what he was doing, resulting in a clamp being placed across the neck of the aneurysm. This cut off the blood supply to the whole of Tristan's lower body, including his kidneys and his bowel, and the bleeding stopped. The tap had been turned off. Within an hour, the diseased piece of aorta was replaced with a material graft before Tristan's wounds were stitched back together.

Although the surgical instruments had been put away and the theatre team could take a rest, Tristan's illness was only just beginning. His lungs had become filled with fluid, preventing him from safely being taken off the life-support machine. An X-ray of his chest showed large fluffy white areas where his black air-filled lungs should have been. This was due to the large volume of blood and fluids that were transfused during the operation, along with his body's inflammatory reaction to major surgery. The extra clotting products that were used – found in normal blood but deficient from stored blood transfusions – also contained white immune blood cells that were reacting to Tristan's tissues and causing a transfusion-related acute lung injury.

Tristan's heart was also weak. Vascular disease is rarely limited to just one area of the body. It was likely that the same disease processes that had caused Tristan's aorta to rupture were also occurring in the blood vessels around his heart and brain. To keep up with the demands of critical illness, his heart was now working as hard as if he were running a marathon without the benefit of health, training or youth.

In addition, the amount of urine draining into Tristan's catheter bag had been decreasing every hour since the operation. While the stress of surgery can cause this to happen naturally through the release of antidiuretic hormone, it was rarely to this extent. A blood test on his kidneys confirmed that Tristan had developed kidney failure. The blood-thinning medication that would usually be administered in order for the kidney machine to be used posed too great a risk of Tristan bleeding. Instead, large amounts of citrate were circulated around the pipes of the machine. This citrate binds calcium, an essential element needed to form blood clots, thereby preventing any clots from forming in the circuit. Without this, blood clots forming in the tubes of the machine would have created a serious blockage.

Although we had machines and drugs to help with these problems, we were most worried about the blood we saw in Tristan's stools. The surgical clamp that had saved his life during the operation had also stopped the blood supply to his bowel. The aneurysm had been repaired, but lack of blood supply to his bowel may have continued, causing the tissue to slowly die and bleed. While the risks were high, there was little option other than to retrace the journey from the ICU back to the emergency theatre for Mr Ruddle to remove the parts of Tristan's bowel that were dying from lack of blood supply.

Critical minutes turned into hours, and hours into days for Tristan. I tell families that the road to recovery from a completely critical illness is always longer than they think. Even the youngest, fittest of patients with a reversible illness can take months to return to a functional normal. Although Tristan had survived the onslaught of problems from his two emergency operations, he was weak. He needed a tracheotomy to wean from the ventilator, his kidneys had only just started working, and he needed extra nutrition through fluid into his veins as his remaining bowel struggled to cope.

With the help of the ICU staff, Mr Ruddle took Tristan outside into the autumn sunshine, still attached to the ventilator, twenty-eight days after he had picked him up in his surf van. Tristan sat in the hospital garden, listening to the breeze and watching the leaves move. Although still very ill, he was able to communicate, able to smile while watching his favourite television programmes and able to see his family again. He also could tell the team what he did and didn't want should his condition worsen. Although Tristan lacked his physical independence, he did regain this mental independence. When his illness progressed, he died peacefully in the manner of his choosing. We didn't prevent death, but we did prolong a life with meaning, with choices and with dignity. And that was a good in itself.

The operation was not the last contribution that the vascular surgery team would make to patients like Tristan. Led by Mr Ruddle's surgical colleague Mr Hedges, the team soon piloted a new screening programme for aneurysms, which invited selected healthy people with risk factors to have a painless ultrasound scan of their aorta. Those found to have an aneurysm were offered a planned surgical repair under controlled, ideal circumstances before it grew too large and too dangerous. The success of this and other screening programmes led to its expansion nationwide and is estimated to have halved the number of deaths from ruptured aneurysms.

9

THE SOUL

Death lives on

Death is something we deal with frequently in intensive care. Overall, one in five patients admitted will die, often in a relatively controlled fashion after further treatment has been deemed no longer in the patient's best interests. At this point, we direct care towards treating pain and distress while stopping treatments that no longer offer any benefit. This will normally result in the patient dying, surrounded by loved ones. We shouldn't hang our heads in shame at this. Intensive care medicine is not always about epic saves and hi-tech, life-saving wizardry. It is also about compassion, about honesty, about making cups of tea for grieving relatives, about reminiscing over good times with them and acknowledging that life is precious. Death is not always a failure; sometimes it is a fitting end to a life well lived. We are experts at saving lives yet also passionate about letting go in the best possible way we can.

My career began with an early introduction to this process. As a young doctor, I was delighted to start working in a friendly, supportive hospital in the small town of Bridgend, South Wales. Sadly, my time there coincided with a spate of teenage suicides in the local community. The boys and girls who were found before death were brought to our intensive care unit. There started the difficult and soon-familiar process of assessing their neurological outcome. All of them died. A total of twenty young people, with their lives ahead of them, died through hanging in just three months, with twenty families left grieving. In the ICU, we see the sharp side of the global mental-health crisis. I worry that this reflects an area of medicine that struggles for funding, recognition and public awareness. I have a plea: to those suffering, please talk to others; to those in positions empowered to help, please listen.

We are also passionate about not travelling down a futile path if adequate warning is given. Accepting death is never easy. Today, one in three patients with terminal cancer will die following an intensive care admission. These are patients expected, predicted, predetermined to die. Yet they do so following medical interventions, surrounded by machines as well as their families. This has been shown to cause more pain and more distress and to incur more costs than effective palliative care.

Peering over the brink of life can be a heavy burden for those trying to pull patients back and I have personally known three colleagues who have themselves stumbled into the dark, joining their past patients who have died. Doctors are twice as likely as all other professions to kill themselves, with a staggering one in twenty-five doctors' deaths being attributable to suicide. This figure grows even greater for doctors facing patient complaints.

Colleagues of mine who have died appeared to be the happiest, most carefree and stable people on the outside. We are taught to cope, to wear a cloak of resilience when speaking to relatives, but this disguise can also prevent others from recognising the help we need. We find it hard to ever forgive ourselves for errors that we have made. These errors are not worn on our sleeves, but we feel them inside. We face the stigma of mental illness even within healthcare, compounded by personal problems to battle just as others face in all walks of life.

Personally, I find sudden, unpredictable death the most difficult to resolve. During a run of busy winter weekend shifts, I was caring for a lady called Patricia who was in her mid-eighties. Although she had been very unwell, her illness had improved to the extent that she was waiting to move to a normal hospital ward. She had a strong personality, knew what she wanted and what she needed, and was happy to tell the staff if things were not to her liking. Yet Patricia had a sparkle in her eyes that meant she was loved by everyone. One day, I overheard her talking about her past life as a dancer with the Tiller Girls in the 1950s. When I asked about her fascinating life, she encouraged me to buy a book she had written entitled *The Girl in the Spotty Dress*.

I ordered her book that lunchtime after reading the

blurb, which summarised Patricia's journey to the peak of her fame. The book's cover featured the iconic photograph of her wearing a vibrant red-spotted dress (Appendix: Figure 5), and she remained instantly recognisable from that original image with the sparkle in her eyes in no way diminished. Patricia made me promise to bring in the book after that weekend so that she could sign it. I was delighted when the book dropped through my letterbox on Monday morning, and I strolled onto the ICU with it firmly clutched in hand and my pen signature-ready. Unfortunately, Patricia had died suddenly late on Sunday night before she had the chance to sign it, and instead I found myself signing her death certificate on that Monday morning. Some months later, I read in the local newspaper that Patricia had been buried in her red spotty dress. I smiled and then I cried.

~

Knowing whether you are doing well at work is so fundamental that it seldom needs stating. If you work in business, you may focus on monthly sales figures and financial targets. Those in customer-service roles use customer satisfaction surveys as a benchmark. In healthcare, surgeons see their patients months after an operation, hoping to hear how the knife has improved their lives. Family doctors experience decades-long patient relationships that have many ups as well as downs.

The feedback I get at work is rather more immediate. I get satisfaction from seeing patients improve over seconds, minutes and hours during the course of a shift. I feel their skin turn from cold and clammy to warm and dry after giving them powerful drugs. I see flashing bright monitors with numbers changing every second as they move into the normal range before I can go home feeling content. In the longer term, I follow up patients to see whether they got better and made it to the general wards or whether they died.

I do occasionally see patients after leaving the ICU. Some return and leave kind gifts or shakily handwritten cards filled with hope about the future and praise for the past. But the greatest privilege – one that extinguishes the burning ember of medical burnout in an instant – is to visit a patient back in their own home. Working in intensive care brings tough times but they can be forgotten in the blink of an eye when I shake the strong hand of a patient I thought was going to die. Nothing compares – no big city job with a fast car, no transient joy after hitting your Christmas bonus, and no early finish on a sunny Friday afternoon. The lives our machines and our staff save are all around us, walking, talking, smiling, and living another day in the sun. I was lucky to visit Joe at home when he was still recovering from his severe brain injury. He was both the same as I remembered yet different. While he had previously been a temporary presence in my world of numbers and science, I was now entering his actual life. This was a rare pleasure.

Happily, intensive care follow-up clinics are being introduced in some hospitals to make this feedback more common. These outpatient clinics invite certain people back after their critical illness to talk through their experiences and ongoing issues. Many will describe problems that are poorly appreciated, such as sleep disturbance, hair loss, low libido and dry skin – ailments that are a world away from the illnesses patients have recovered from, but still of huge personal importance. Small numbers of survivors will reveal symptoms of post-traumatic stress, including flashbacks as severe as those of soldiers returning from war. Voice problems are also common, especially in patients who needed a tracheotomy, and some will experience swallowing difficulties. These clinics are extremely important; however, they miss an important section of patients that we have cared for: those who didn't make it.

~

Ten years after Christopher died following his admission to intensive care with sepsis, I went to visit his family to ask them about the aftermath of his death. Simply writing to them after this period of time was one of the hardest things I've ever done – I was extremely worried about asking them to relive a painful past. At the same time, I feel strongly that families and patients should at least be given the opportunity to tell their story and I hoped that offering to recount their story would not only help them, but also help others.

Entering through the colourful glass front door, it was clear that life had stood still for Christopher's family since the day he died. His mum talked bravely and openly about how the experience of Christopher's illness still weighs heavily on her and her family even a decade later. She was pleased when Christopher's suffering eventually ended but distraught that this meant losing her eighteen-year-old son.

The level of detail Christopher's family gave about the events in 2009 was remarkable. Their pain had been etched into an indelible record, glazed by the love they had and the loss they felt. The smells of the hospital were still stuck in their noses, the colours of the relatives' room they sat in for hours still make them sad. Hearing this level of honesty reminds me how important it is to get things right for families, especially when giving bad news. Having a fleck of blood on your shoe or wrongly pronouncing a patient's name are among things I am embarrassed to have done after long night shifts. For a mum or a dad or a sister, these oversights will stay with them for ever.

A striking theme that reoccurs when speaking with families is the reluctance of others to acknowledge death. In the days after his son's death, Christopher's dad saw old friends and colleagues. Most would physically avoid him in the street or even look the other way while passing on an escalator simply so as not to confront his loss. The medicalisation of death over the last hundred years has had a huge impact on how we deal with death and how we grieve. Today few people have seen someone die and even fewer have spent time with the dead. Think back to the last time you were told that a friend's mum, dad or child had died. The standard response is to say: 'Oh, I'm so sorry,' before offering some kind of practical or emotional help. You then may try to find a way out of the situation as quickly as possible.

After talking to Christopher's family, I now do the exact opposite. People enjoy talking about those they love and why should this change after they die? This desire may even grow stronger. If you were to tell me that your mum had recently died, I would now instead ask you questions about her: 'What was her name? What was she like? What did she look like? What did she enjoy doing when she was alive? What song did you play at her funeral?' After death, I now ask about life. I encourage you to do so too.

Talking about death and breaking bad news should be a core skill for any intensive care doctor. We will have, on average, more than 200 difficult conversations every year, telling families that their loved ones may die or will never be the same again. Incrementally, each conversation takes its toll, saying sorry, watching other people cry with hope and fear. All in the knowledge that one day, that will be you.

I have told a mother that her son has died, a son that his father has killed his mother, fiancés that their weddings need to be cancelled, and husbands of fifty years that they can never say sorry for that last silly argument they had with their beloved wife. We carry these people and their stories around with us, long after the graves have been filled or the ashes scattered.

The reactions of a family to bad news are equally as broad as the tragedies involved. People cry, scream, laugh, run away, thank us, understand, hit the wall and hit themselves. They beg us to be wrong, they deny death is actually possible, and even the atheist can plead to various gods for a miracle. These reactions are not right or wrong, they are just part of human grief and the sacrifice needed to make love possible. A heart can break only if it has first loved.

It is important to use the right language in medicine especially when a patient has actually died. The power of disbelief during grief will make families interpret your words in the way that is least painful for them. 'I'm afraid we have lost your mum' or, 'Your dad is no longer with us' or, 'Your son has gone to a better place' will be interpreted literally. 'Where have they gone?' comes the reply. Instead, I confront reality and now say: 'I'm very sorry but they have died.'

Each difficult conversation is difficult in its own way, although there is a similar process I go through each time – perhaps selfishly to help me more than others. This process starts with getting to really know the story. For me, getting the personal details right, knowing what jobs they do, what their beliefs are, shows a straightforward respect for others. And so I reread the patient notes, know their story inside out and then put their hospital sticker on the palm of my left hand with the nurse's name handwritten in the corner. A quick glance before meeting the family reminds my busy brain of the names I must not get wrong.

Next comes the environment. Relatives' rooms in a cash-strapped health system are difficult to prioritise when the money is hardly enough to pay for nurses and pillows. This fails to recognise the importance of a family's lasting memories of the moment they were told the worst news of their lives. Having a nice pair of curtains will not dull the pain of losing someone but having blood on the floor, a broken, draughty window and nowhere to sit certainly can make it even more difficult.

I am lucky to know an inspirational lady, Rhian Mannings Burke, who turned her family tragedy into a way to help others. When her son George was just one year, one week and one day old, he died from severe infection. In the cold, mint-white, clinical environment of the emergency department, Rhian carried her dead son down the corridor, past onlookers, to find privacy in an unused office where she could spend time with George, surrounded by flashing screensavers and Post-it notes on the walls. Racked with grief, her husband Paul died five days later. Rather than allow these unimaginable events to destroy her, Rhian redirected her emotions towards helping others. She founded the charity 2 Wish Upon A Star, which builds thoughtful family rooms in hospitals, ideally designed for breaking bad news, complete with bereavement boxes that allow lasting memories to be made from handprints and hair cuttings after sudden death. When I sit in our relatives' room today, it is thanks to Rhian's strength that families have a better experience than she once had.

I like to check the room before families enter, quickly removing any paraphernalia of grief that has been left behind, putting my phone on silent and ensuring my appearance is appropriate. The little things matter. Families meet around ten new people every day during a typical intensive care stay and so, despite name badges, we must remember to introduce ourselves each time we meet. As I sit down next to the family with the patient's nurse, I say: 'Hello. I am Matt Morgan, one of the intensive care consultants,' before asking the family to introduce themselves. I never miss out this step after learning from my earlier toe-curling mistakes of calling a daughter a wife and even a husband a daughter. Then comes a warning shot: 'I'm sorry to say that this is going to be a very difficult conversation. I don't have any good news to tell you, I'm afraid.'

The amount of information relayed to families, even in these short meetings, can be vast. The amount received, understood and remembered is always significantly smaller, so it is important to ascertain what the family already knows before launching into further details. Despite being unconscious or even dead, confidentiality remains with the patient. Thus, great care is needed when discussing sensitive diagnoses, including HIV infection and cancers that have spread.

After the medical details have been discussed, I like to cover three other aspects. The first is hidden guilt. This can play a huge role in family distress, with relatives feeling 'if only' they had done something differently, their loved one would not be so ill. I address this head-on, especially in the case of cardiac arrests where family members have done CPR. I will say with sincerity: 'If it wasn't for your actions and your care, we wouldn't be here at all right now. You have done everything right. Please remember that.'

The second aspect is that I always give families at least three opportunities to ask questions at different points in the conversation. I only stop saying, 'Are there any other questions I can answer?' when it is followed by a long, hanging silence.

The third comes at the end of a conversation, when I ask families something that seems difficult and uncomfortable. I say, gesturing to an empty chair: 'If your dad was sitting here now, listening to us speak, what would he say?' Replies can often be light-hearted, with families saying with a smile: 'Oh, he was such a joker, he probably would have said something funny!' I use this question as a way to gain a subtle insight into the person I have been treating but may never properly meet. It can also offer families added psychological permission to express opinions they may not feel comfortable saying in their own voice. Stepping meta-phorically into the role of your loved one may open up new avenues of thought. Families will often reply with such profound statements as: 'He would say: "Don't resuscitate me" or, "Just let me go."' Admitting this as a grieving wife can be impossible but saying it as someone you respect and love can be just a little easier.

~

I have some bad news. You are going to die. So am I. So are we all. Derren Brown's excellent book *Happy* summarises the benefits of this when he says: 'Death, perhaps uniquely among objects of our dread, instructs us how to live.' What is important, therefore, is what we have done in life, how we have treated others and what we leave behind.

After meeting Christopher's family a decade after his death, it was clear that he had left a lot. With the proceeds from charity events after his funeral, his family supported one of the things that Christopher had most cherished during his time in Africa. He had walked with children from a local slum to the top of Mount Kenya, speaking to them about their hopes for the future. With no school, no money and no family, the children's hopes were ironically the same as Christopher's would become: to survive. Six months after his death, the money raised was spent building a new school, brick by brick, on the outskirts of Nairobi. This gave hope to those same children to thrive and not simply survive. Today you can visit the school, which bears a plaque engraved with Christopher's favourite song, 'Don't Worry Be Happy'. Ten years since his death, there are now children from those slums working in the very hospital in Nairobi where Christopher was cared for.

His legacy goes further than that. It was thanks to Christopher that I became involved with pressure groups to raise awareness of sepsis as the killer of more people every year than breast, lung and prostate cancer combined. The work of the UK Sepsis Trust and the Global Sepsis Alliance has resulted in improved sepsis care worldwide, focusing on early antibiotic use and governmental support. Their 'Think Sepsis' campaign aims to alert the public to early symptoms of this devastating disease. Thousands of people are alive today as a result of the impact that Christopher had on the people around him.

~

In Chapter 6 we met Steven, who had recently become a father just five months before his admission to intensive care. We left his story as it started, with his skin being warm to the touch, even though he had died. How was this possible?

Surprisingly, there is no official definition of death in British law. Instead, we have a number of guidelines including that from the Academy of Medical Royal Colleges, which states:

Death entails the irreversible loss of those essential characteristics which are necessary to the existence of a living human person and, thus, the definition of death should be regarded as the irreversible loss of the capacity for consciousness, combined with irreversible loss of the capacity to breathe.

When I am called to see a patient who has died, I perform the same ritual each time. Firstly, I talk to the dead. Whenever I meet patients in intensive care, they often have their eyes closed, either due to sedation or their illness. I still talk to them and explain what I am doing. We are often surprised in the weeks and months after recovery how snippets of conversations can be recalled even by our sickest patients. Therefore, communication is as important as ever. For me, this human respect extends after death even though no conversations will ever be recounted.

I say hello and introduce myself. I tell them that I am going to feel their pulse as I press my index and middle fingers on the side of their neck to feel for the characteristic tapping of the carotid artery. At the same time, I place my stethoscope onto their chest to listen for the *lub-dub* sound of the heart valves. Then I wait. I wait a long, silent, slow five minutes. I listen for silence and feel for the presence of absence. No sound is heard and no pulse is felt.

I then open the eyes of the patient, shine my pen torch into the depths of the black pupils. In life the pupils would respond by tightening to a mere speck of black, but not after death. They remain as large, dark windows, no longer looking out yet still allowing light to fall in. Finally, I press firmly on the bony ridge above the eye after saying: 'I'm sorry.' Nothing happens. The patient is dead. Doing the same to Steven, even after his severe brain bleed, I could feel his pulse and hear his heart beat. Yet he too was dead.

In 1976, a series of tests on the brain was ratified to indicate that further medical treatment would be futile. Three years later these brainstem tests were unified with the concept of death so that patients fulfilling these criteria were dead.

The brainstem is a 7 cm elongation between the brain and spinal cord, divided into the midbrain, pons and medulla. Despite its small size, it is the motherboard of the brain and of the person. It is integral to the essential functions of life including breathing, coughing, metabolic control and heart rate. Without a functioning brainstem, life is simply not possible.

Due to the location of this structure, excess pressure in any part of the brain can result in brainstem failure. Transmitted pressure due to disease will attempt to extrude the brain through any orifice available. The large exit at the bottom of the skull, the foramen magnum, is the obvious choice. The brainstem is thus squeezed through a narrowing too small to be accommodated. A lack of blood supply ensues, followed by lack of oxygen and cell death in the brainstem.

For Steven, as we could not fix his problems, the trajectory of his life was already laid out in front of him. The blood inside his head from the ruptured aneurysm increased the pressure in his brain and blocked the small channels where spinal fluid normally flowed. This led to further increases in pressure as spinal fluid accumulated in his ventricles. This forced the brainstem downwards against the hard ridge around the edges of his foramen magnum. At first, blood failed to get to the outer surface of the brainstem, causing huge fluctuations in blood pressure and an erratic heart rate. Next, the circuits that controlled Steven's eye reflexes failed. When we shone a light into his eyes, his big, black pupils did not shrink. Then, the wiring that transmitted sensations of pain from his body to his brain was damaged. Pressing hard on his eyebrow no longer led to a reaction. The same damage occurred in the nerves controlling his cough reflex, his gag reflex, his balance centre, and even his ability to blink. Then the breathing centre in the medulla failed, meaning Steven would never again have the urge to breathe.

As a colleague spoke to Steven's partner about our worst fears, I prepared the equipment needed to conduct formal brainstem testing. The procedure we followed is logical, structured, and carried out on two entirely separate occasions by only the most highly qualified of doctors. It is something I take very seriously and do with utmost respect.

We first ensured that certain preconditions were met. We checked that no drugs had been used that might impact upon the results. We checked Steven's hormone system was working sufficiently, ensured his temperature was normal and looked in detail at all of his brain scans. We proceeded through a series of tests to ensure that the function of nine of the twelve essential brainstem nerves that can be tested had failed. These nerve failures explained the problems we had already noted, including why Steven's eyes no longer reacted to light and why he no longer coughed. As I tested each nerve, my colleague independently observed for any responses. Only if we both agreed unequivocally would that particular criterion be fulfilled. Steven failed all nine of the nerve tests.

We then moved on to the second stage of testing, where Steven's life-support machine was disconnected entirely for five long, silent minutes. We looked closely at Steven's chest and abdomen every second, trying to observe any breathing. At the same time, we delivered enough oxygen via a thin tube placed into his lungs to prevent any damage to his body from a lack of oxygen. Steven did not breathe at all in that long five-minute period. It was 10.34 p.m. when the first set of tests were complete. My colleague and I both sat down, had a drink of water and then returned to do the tests all over again.

The second set of tests confirmed what we found during the first set. No case of recovery has ever been reported after an appropriately conducted process of brainstem death testing. 10.34 p.m. will be a time etched into Steven's history for ever. It is the time of completion of the first set of brainstem tests. In law, it is the time when Steven died. What his family did next is remarkable.

After the second set of brainstem tests had been completed, Steven's family gathered in our relatives' room. Its walls are saturated with words of sadness, family tears, loss and anger. Cradled by her family, Steven's partner had guessed what was coming. Relatives often understand and predict bad news long before we are even sure of it ourselves. My colleague Dr Hingston delicately explained that we had conducted two sets of detailed tests. As a result of his bleed, Steven had fulfilled all of the criteria for brainstem death. After the first tear fell from Steven's partner's cheek, she asked: 'Can he help someone else?'

The legislation surrounding organ donation in Wales changed just prior to Steven's death. It had moved from an opt-in process to an opt-out scheme where consent for donation after death was presumed. Although this doesn't negate the need for family assent, it has brought the issue squarely into the public consciousness, which is perhaps its greatest benefit.

Brainstem death allows patients the opportunity to donate their organs under ideal conditions. Those who have already died according to brainstem-testing criteria are able to donate their organs through a well-planned, organised and calm operation that maintains blood flow to the tissues until the very last moment. This gives recipients the best chance of having a life-changing donation that will function well. It is the greatest gift anyone could ever give.

Steven's family were given as much time as they needed to talk through their wishes with a specialist team. However, their bravery didn't stop there. A documentary film was being made at the time to raise public awareness of the organ donation legislation changes in Wales. Steven's partner, with great strength, dignity and thought for others, allowed their experiences as a family to be filmed in real time. Twelve months later, the BBC documentary *The Greatest Gift* was watched by nearly half a million people. It showed, for the first time, the process of brainstem testing, with myself and Dr Hingston explaining the science behind its use to viewers. The series has been awarded a BAFTA in recognition of not only the way in which it handled a difficult subject, but the ongoing contribution it will make to the public understanding of medicine.

Twenty four hours after Steven died, his gift had allowed three other patients to live: a man who has since travelled the world with Steven's liver inside him, a lady who had struggled on a kidney-transplant waiting list for years, and a child who now has a piece of Steven's heart inside of their own. Look at your closest loved one right now – maybe your son or daughter, your mum or your dad. Imagine the feeling should the phone ring offering them another chance at life through the gift of donation from someone just like Steven. Imagine that same phone call saying that the gift has instead been cremated or buried. Donation is not only the greatest gift that can be given, but it is a gift that is of no value unless it *is* given. Intensive care medicine facilitates this most selfless human act. We care for the physical body of a patient, even after their soul has departed. We protect their organs, ensuring their donation has the maximum benefit to recipients who may live hundreds of miles away. Although these people will never have met the donor, their second shot at life can be a constant reminder to us all of how far humanity and medicine have come.

I hope that Chapter 4 can save a life through teaching CPR. I hope this chapter can save more lives if just one of you considers what you leave behind after your death. Think about how what you no longer need could transform the lives of others. Once you have thought about this, no matter the outcome, tell your family about your wishes. Death need not detract from the joy of living. Even in death you can leave a legacy of hope for others, just like Steven and Christopher.

EPILOGUE

Work hard, ask questions and be nice

There are two questions that I am asked most commonly. The first is: 'How do you deal with the stress?' This is closely followed by: 'How do you switch off?' Although I normally offer an easy answer, such as I enjoy running or reading, the truth is far more complex. I was recently working when a severely injured nineteen-year-old cyclist was brought to the ICU. She was a student and had been hit at high speed by a van while riding home after lectures. She was critically ill with a traumatic brain injury, a pelvic fracture and multiple chest injuries. It took hours of work for our team to stabilise her condition, which involved performing difficult, bloody, practical procedures, co-ordinating multiple surgical specialists and speaking to her distraught family.

That evening, I inevitably left work late and cycled myself the nine miles home along narrow country lanes towards the Welsh coast. During the journey, my mind continuously replayed sections of the day that had gone well and others that could have gone better. I thought about the ensuing dramatic changes to that poor young student's life, and I thought about her family. I worried about my safety when braking around a few tight corners. That day was challenging and stressful, but for me it was not unmanageably stressful in an obvious sense. Often, the medical part of the job is actually the least stressful aspect. Visiting patients as part of my research for this book years after I had first cared for them has brought some of the most nerve-wrecking moments I have faced in my career – often more so than when I was their doctor.

For me, stress is trying to perform when you lack control, training or resources. It is when lots of small problems arrive all at the same time. It is when disorder reigns. Looking after that nineteen-year-old cyclist, I had control, the right training and adequate resources. Stress in medicine often comes in a slowly increasing gradient, over years not seconds, sometimes hardly noticeable until it becomes too much. It comes when the system places demands that you want to meet but are unable to. As soon as my cycle ride home ended, I became stressed. I returned home to a situation where I had little control, no training and few resources. Dismounting from my bike after that long day, I stepped through the gate into my neighbour's back garden where I was responsible for the health of his prized cucumbers for the duration of his holiday. As I opened his greenhouse door, still wearing my hospital badge, things got worse. Half of the leaves on the cucumber plants were not as green and vibrant as they had been when he showed me around. Instead, they were dry, crispy and covered in white spots. The cucumbers were dying and I did not know what to do.

Odd though it sounds, for me this was the stressful part of my day. This is not to downplay the enormity of the young cyclist's injuries in any way. But in that greenhouse I lacked control, insight and a team around me. I didn't have the knowledge or the skills to deal with what was ahead of me. I couldn't speak to my neighbour. I couldn't ask for help. Yes, intensive care medicine can be hard, and at night when I close my eyes I am often troubled by thoughts of patients past and present who have lived and died. But that is my work and that is my life and that is my choice. And here lies the key not only to intensive care but to medicine as a whole. I work in a system that is imperfect. Stress occurs and relationships break down when the system is stretched. When the system is stressed, so am I. This is often not due to the inherent nature of the work, but to the inherent nature of the imperfect system. As long as those who work in the health system are being looked after, then being an intensive care doctor doesn't need to be the most stressful job in the world. However, the ongoing pressures on the NHS mean that health workers, including myself, sometimes *don't* feel looked after. Look after the system and you will look after its workers. Look after the workers and they will look after the patients.

～

I feel uncomfortable about the number of times that the word 'I' has been used in this book. This book is not about me but about patients. It must, of course, be told through the prism of my personal experience, hence my indulgence in letting you peer into how patients have touched my career and my life. But within this book's story of the specialty of critical care and the wonderful profession of medicine, I am the least important person – not least because there are thousands of people just like me all around the world, doing bigger and better things right now.

I do not always lead. I cannot always lead. Sometimes I want someone to throw out a thick rope and haul me in. Being an assistant for much of our lives is not something to be ashamed of – followership is as essential as leadership. This is as true when I head home and become a follower of my children, my spouse or our dog. Good leaders should know when to lead and, more importantly, when to shut up and listen. Our hospital doctors, porters, surgeons and cleaners are all educated, expected to problem-solve and to be able to influence or to disrupt. They are not passive subordinates. We should equally celebrate and cherish those who deliver unglamorous help to those most in need.

Although each story I have told is special, even more remain untold. I am privileged that writing this book has allowed the best job in the world to now also be the best life in the world, allowing me to travel, speak and write to you. I have been eagerly waiting for the opportunity to tell others what intensive care medicine can do and how it does it. I am delighted that Mrs Robertson, my careers advisor, did not have a satisfactory answer when I told her, aged fifteen, that I wanted to be Fox Mulder from *The X-Files*. Medicine was a much better, although more dangerous, choice. Thank you, Mrs Robertson.

The job we do is hard but I love this job often because it *is* hard. Sometimes doing the hard thing is an easy decision, and that decision is made even easier by the amazing team of people I work with each and every day. Thank you to the NHS, the cleaners, the canteen workers, the nurses and the porters, the doctors and the physiotherapists.

When these people all come together, amazing things can happen.

Intensive care is not always about fancy machines. It is not always about the great save. It is not even always about medicine. This was clear today more than ever as colleagues from our intensive care unit organised a wedding for a patient who had remained critically ill for over a year. Too ill to leave hospital, the wedding came to him as he married his long-term partner of over thirty years surrounded by staff who had become good friends. Finally, if I could offer just one piece of advice to those considering a career in intensive care it would be to work hard, ask questions and be kind to people. It is the best job in the world.

APPENDIX OF FIGURES

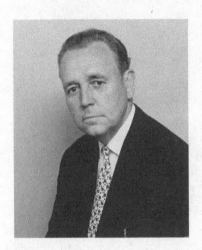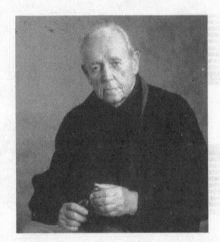

Figure 1: Dr Bjorn Ibsen, aged thirty-five in 1950 (left), and shortly before his death aged ninety-one in 2007 (right). Although he often attributed his success to chance and coincidence, he was a strong person with a healthy degree of self-belief. Following the polio outbreak, he was awarded the Danish poliomyelitis medal, the anaesthetic medal and the Purkinje medal from Czechoslovakia. He wrote a number of books, including two intensive care medicine textbooks and a memoir entitled *The Happiness of Reunions*.

(Credit: Medical Museion, University of Copenhagen)

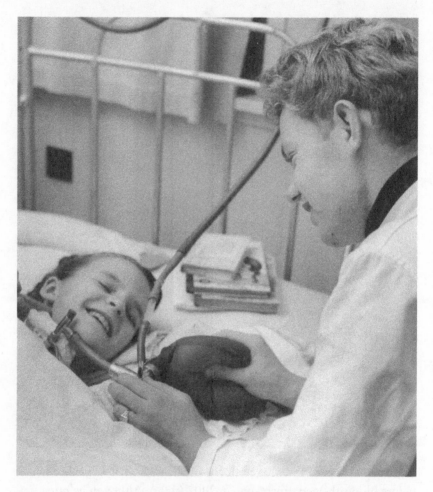

Figure 2: A medical student keeping a little girl alive by squeezing a bag attached to her tracheotomy during the Copenhagen polio epidemic. It is unclear whether this is Vivi, although it does bear a striking resemblance, with some of her favourite books laid on her pillow.

(Credit: Medical Museion, University of Copenhagen)

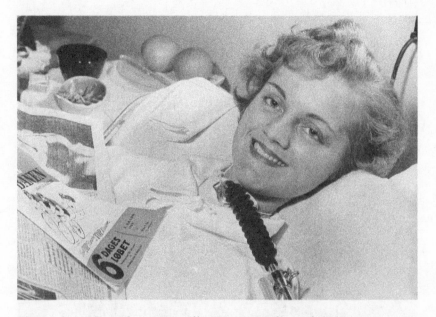

Figure 3: Vivi, aged twenty, still enjoying reading while living at home with her mum. In the background can be seen some food items that she was still able to eat despite her tracheotomy and the power lead connected to her portable ventilator.

(Credit: Sven Riedel)

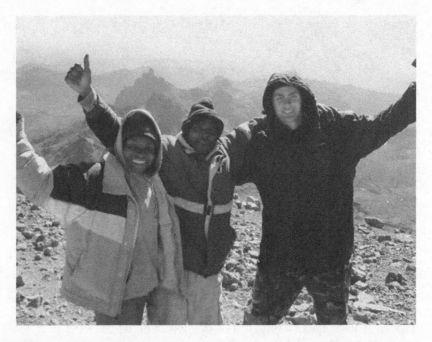

Figure 4: Christopher at the top of Mount Kenya, shortly before he became unwell, accompanied by some local children. After his death, the money raised by his family would build a school to offer these children a better future.

(Photo courtesy of Christopher's family)

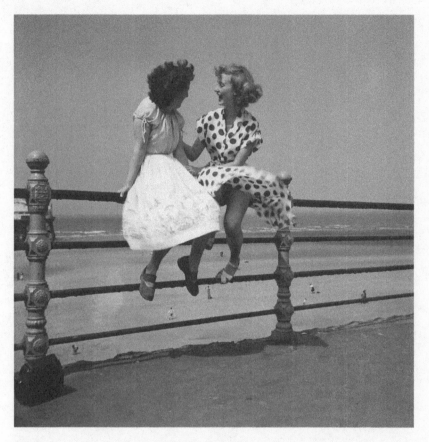

Figure 5: 'The Girl in the Spotty Dress'. The iconic photo of Patricia (right) on Blackpool North Pier in 1951. Following her death, she was buried wearing that same spotted dress.

(Credit: Getty Images)

ACKNOWLEDGEMENTS

Firstly, thank you to Charlotte, my wonderful literary agent, who took a chance on an unpublished stranger. Thank you to my fantastic editors, Fritha Saunders, Charlotte Atyeo and Melissa Bond. Thank you to my mum and dad for their unwavering support and encouragement. Thank you to my wife, Alison, and my two daughters, Evie and Amelia, for giving me the greatest reasons for coming home after a hard day's work. But most of all, thank you to the patients who lived whom I shall remember for a very long time, and to those patients who died whom I shall remember for ever.

This book has been written in countless cities, countries and time zones. It has been fuelled by a never-ending stream of coffees and pains aux raisins. Three places deserve a special mention. Pete and his team in The Plug coffee shop have made my life significantly better. The comfy chair in Academy Espresso has been gifted a perfect impression of my imperfect bottom. On my laptop is a beautiful piece of software, Ulysses, that has kept me typing for over 70,000 words, occasionally while sitting in the greatest bar on earth, Scarfes Bar in London.

Thank you to Dr Anders Perner, Sven Riedel, Sussi Bokelund Hansen and Nana Bokelund Kroon for their help in tracing Vivi's story, and to Dr Julie Highfield for her invaluable advice on contacting patients. The PhD thesis of Dr Louise Reisner-Sénélar from Goethe University Frankfurt was also enormously helpful. Dr Peter Brindley has been a hugely important writing companion and Laura Prosser has improved both my health through her physical coaching and this book through her attention to detail. Thanks to the BMJ publishing group and Dr Mark Taubert, who allowed me to reproduce elements of my online blog. Thank you to Christopher's family, Getty Images, Sven Riedel and the Medical Museion at the University of Copenhagen for their images. Thank you to the many mentors I have had over the years, especially Dr Gary Thomas, Dr Mathias Eberl and Dr Matt Wise. Finally, thank you to the numerous people from the medical community who read early drafts, including Cai Gwinnut, Stephen Leadbeatter, Steve Edlin, Anna Batchelor and Farhad Kapadia.

References

Preface

p.xii   'Although one in five of you admitted will eventually die in an intensive care unit, many of you won't even know what that is.' Garcia-Labattut A *et al.* [Degree of public awareness regarding intensive care units (ICUs) and intensive care physicians in Castilla y Leon]. *Med Intensiva.* 2006 Mar;30(2):45–51.

1: An Introduction to the World of Intensive Care Medicine

p.3   'with 130 people dying as a result.' Lassen, H. C. A. The Epidemic of Poliomyelitis in Copenhagen, 1952. *Proceedings of the Royal Society of Medicine* 47, 67–71 (1954).

p.5   'This was the world's first intensive care unit, requiring over 1,500 volunteer medical students to squeeze Vivi's bag and then the bags of countless other patients day in, day out for six months during the Copenhagen polio epidemic.' Trubuhovich, R. V. The 1952–1953 Danish epidemic of poliomyelitis and Bjorn Ibsen. *Crit Care Resusc* 5, 312 (2003).

p.7   'It should contain 10 per cent of the total number of beds in the hospital and be located close to the operating theatres and the emergency department.' Sasabuchi, Y. *et al.* The Volume-Outcome Relationship in Critically Ill Patients in Relation to the ICU-to-Hospital Bed Ratio. *Critical Care Medicine* 43 (2015).

p.7   'We can classify the severity of a patient's illness throughout the hospital – and the subsequent care that they need – into five different levels from 0 to 4.' The Intensive Care Society. Levels of Critical Care for Adult Patients. 1–12 (2009).

p.9   'It is no wonder that we intensive care doctors feel unsure of ourselves when expected to assimilate the 13,000 diagnoses, 6,000 drugs and 4,000 surgical procedures …' Fitzpatrick, L. Atul Gawande: How to Make Doctors Better. *Time* (2010).

p.10   'The cream contained aspirin as the active ingredient, the willow-bark extract originally used by ancient Egyptians as a remedy for aches and pains.' Vainio, H. & Morgan, G. Aspirin for the second hundred years: new uses for an old drug. *Pharmacol. Toxicol.* 81, 151–152 (1997).

p.16   'Atul Gawande's paradigm-shifting book, *The Checklist Manifesto.*' Gawande, A. (2010). *The Checklist Manifesto: How To Get Things Right.* New York: Metropolitan Books.

p.16   'His introduction of the World Health Organization's "Surgical Safety Checklist" has saved millions of lives …' Haynes, A. B. *et al.* A surgical safety checklist to reduce morbidity and mortality in a global population. *N Engl J Med* 360, 491–499 (2009).

p.17   '… Nobel Prize-winning Daniel Kahneman in his life-affirming book, *Thinking, Fast and Slow.*' Kahneman, D. (2011). Toronto: Doubleday Canada.

p.18   'Although our research is ongoing …' Clinical Trials Gov. Using Wearable Technology to Predict Perioperative High-Risk Patient Outcomes (STEPS). https://clinicaltrials.gov/ct2/show/NCT03328039 (2018) (Accessed: 22 September 2018).

pp.18–19 'All too often the outcome from this pressurised system, running at nearly 100 per cent capacity, is that operations are frequently postponed.' Wong, D. J. N., Harris, S. K. & Moonesinghe, S. R. Cancelled operations: a 7-day cohort study of planned adult inpatient surgery in 245 UK National Health Service hospitals. *British Journal of Anaesthesia* 121, 730–738 (2018).

p.19   'This simple yet effective strategy has allowed hundreds of operations to proceed in the last year where previously many may have been cancelled.' Cardiff and Vale NHS Trust. 'Bed free ward' in running for national award. http://www.cardiffandvaleuhb.wales.nhs.uk/news/42696 (2016) (Accessed: 22 September 2018).

p.20   '... a single night spent in intensive care costing as much as £3,000.' Halpern, N. A. & Pastores, S. M. Critical care medicine in the United States 2000–2005: An analysis of bed numbers, occupancy rates, payer mix, and costs. *Critical Care Medicine* 38 (2010).

p.20   'For example, analysis suggests that the cost for each additional life saved in intensive care is around £40,000, compared with £220,000 for the treatment of high cholesterol using statins in well patients.' Ridley, S. & Morris, S. Cost effectiveness of adult intensive care in the UK. *Anaesthesia* 62, 547–554 (2007).

p.20   'The average mortality rate for these patients has been incrementally decreasing over time thanks to better systems, better training, better equipment and evidence-based therapies.' Vincent, J.-L. *et al.* Comparison of European ICU patients in 2012 (ICON) versus 2002 (SOAP). *Intensive Care Med* 44, 337–344 (2018).

pp.20–21 'There are now more than 30 million patients admitted to intensive care worldwide every year ...' Extrapolated from Vincent, J.-L. *et al.* International study of the prevalence and outcomes of infection in intensive care units. *JAMA* 302, 2323–2329 (2009).

p.21   'Evidence shows that intensive care is able to significantly increase the chance of survival from critical illness and of leading a meaningful life, not just being alive.' Molina, J. A. D., Seow, E., Heng, B. H., Chong, W. F. & Ho, B. Outcomes of direct and indirect medical intensive care unit admissions from the emergency department of an acute care hospital: a retrospective cohort study. *BMJ Open* 4, e005553 (2014).

2: The Immune System

p.24 'These were the early stages of an infection that had possibly invaded his body during the swim that felt so good at the time.' Tracing the exact moment and place where an infection is contracted is rarely possible. This is one of the plausible explanations and one that Christopher's family feel was most likely.

p.24 '. . . the lungs are by far the most common site of infection.' World Health Organization. *The WHO Global Health Estimates*. WHO (2018).

p.25 'Globally, parasites and helminths (worms) are a significant source of human suffering.' Dagher, G. A., Saadeldine, M., Bachir, R., Zebian, D. & Chebl, R. B. Descriptive analysis of sepsis in a developing country. *International Journal of Emergency Medicine* 8, 19 (2015).

p.25 'In the Western world, it is viruses and bacteria, followed by fungi, that lead to the most problems.' Suarez De La Rica, A., Gilsanz, F. & Maseda, E. Epidemiologic trends of sepsis in western countries. *Annals of Translational Medicine* 4, 325 (2016).

p.26 'This simple classification system has allowed scientists to draw a family tree for different microbe types according to whether they take up the Gram stain, the way that they look microscopically and how they group together.' GRAM, C. Ueber die isolirte Farbung der Schizomyceten in Schnitt-und Trockenpraparaten. *Fortschritte der Medicin* 2, 185–189 (1884).

p.27 '. . . an overwhelming immune response of his body to infection, causing tissue damage and organ failure.' Singer, M. *et al.* The Third International Consensus Definitions for Sepsis and Septic Shock (Sepsis-3). *JAMA* 315, 801–810 (2016).

p.27 'I paused my clinical training to complete a research PhD, attempting to answer the questions that I found myself asking in the wake of Christopher's illness.' Morgan, M. Immune fingerprinting in acute severe sepsis (Cardiff University, 2014).

p.31 'It has been 140 years since the discovery of the germ theory by the German scientist Robert Koch.' Walker, L., Levine, H.

& Jucker, M. Koch's postulates and infectious proteins. *Acta Neuropathol.* 112, 1–4 (2006).

p.32   '... we now have a new method of diagnostic testing for infections.' Zhang, J. *et al.* Machine-learning algorithms define pathogen-specific local immune fingerprints in peritoneal dialysis patients with bacterial infections. *Kidney Int.* 92, 1–13 (2017).

p.33   'It is quite likely that Sam had developed an infection from the chicken she had eaten.' While the infection she developed is typically transmitted through poultry, there are other sources that may have been responsible.

p.34   '... we do know that some people are pre-programmed to be too "hot" and some too "cold".' Petersen, L., Andersen, P. K. & Sørensen, T. I. A. Genetic influences on incidence and case-fatality of infectious disease. *PLoS ONE* 5, e10603 (2010).

p.35   'For example, having the genetic variation BRCA1 leads to a doubling of the risk of developing breast cancer in a woman's lifetime, but around 50 per cent of women with the BRCA1 gene do not develop breast cancer.' Kuchenbaecker, K. B. *et al.* Risks of Breast, Ovarian, and Contralateral Breast Cancer for BRCA1 and BRCA2 Mutation Carriers. *JAMA* 317, 2402–2416 (2017).

p.36   'In a brave series of experiments in 2014, American researchers injected the major component of Gram-negative bacteria cell walls, lipopolysaccharides, into healthy volunteers under close medical supervision.' Dillingh, M. R. *et al.* Characterization of inflammation and immune cell modulation induced by low-dose LPS administration to healthy volunteers. *Journal of Inflammation* 11, 1697 (2014).

p.38   'This would turn out to be the most useful mess in history.' Diggins, F. W. The true history of the discovery of penicillin, with refutation of the misinformation in the literature. *Br J Biomed Sci* 56, 83–93 (1999).

p.38   'This serendipitous mistake would save the lives of around 200 million people globally in the ninety years that followed.' http://www.newworldencyclopedia.org/entry/Alexander_Fleming

p.38   'Anne Miller, a 33-year-old nurse from New York, became the first patient to be treated with this new drug.' Rothman, L. This Is What Happened to the First American Treated With Penicillin. *Time* (2016).

p.40   'They can even be physically passed – through the movement of protein packages called plasmids – to other bacteria that lack these abilities.' Turner, P. E. *et al*. Antibiotic resistance correlates with transmission in plasmid evolution. *Evolution* 68, 3368–3380 (2014).

p.40   'In fact, there has been just one: teixobactin.' Fiers, W. D., Craighead, M. & Singh, I. Teixobactin and Its Analogues: A New Hope in Antibiotic Discovery. *ACS Infect Dis* 3, 688–690 (2017).

p.40   'Antibiotic resistance has been highlighted by the World Health Organization as the most pressing threat to global safety.' https://www.who.int/news-room/fact-sheets/detail/antibiotic-resistance

p.40   '... and international initiatives aim to support the development of new antimicrobial classes.' Kmietowicz, Z. Few novel antibiotics in the pipeline, WHO warns. *BMJ* 358, j4339 (2017).

p.41   '... a delay of just one hour in administration is associated with an increase in the likelihood of death by nearly 8 per cent.' Kumar, A. *et al*. Initiation of inappropriate antimicrobial therapy results in a fivefold reduction of survival in human septic shock. *Chest* 136, 1237–1248 (2009). Although widely quoted, many leading sepsis researchers question this finding. A very good summary of these issues can be found in Singer, M. Antibiotics for Sepsis: Does Each Hour Really Count, or Is It Incestuous Amplification? *American Journal of Respiratory and Critical Care Medicine* 196, 800–802 (2017).

p.42   'Despite these theoretical concerns, international guidelines rightly promote the early administration of antibiotics to those with severe infection, alongside early "source control" where the infectious focus should be removed as quickly as possible.' Singer, M. *et al*. The Third International Consensus Definitions for Sepsis and Septic Shock (Sepsis-3). *JAMA* 315, 801–810 (2016).

p.45   'Occam's razor is a principle much loved in medicine, first
        described by the Franciscan friar William of Ockham.' Whyte,
        M. B. An argument against the use of Occam's razor in modern
        medical education. *Med Teach* 40, 99–100 (2018).

p.48   'The German immunologist and Nobel laureate, Paul Ehrlich,
        coined the term 'horror autotoxicus', or the horror of self-
        toxicity, to describe the body's aversion to immunological
        self-destruction.' Horror Autotoxicus and Other Concepts of
        Paul Ehrlich. *JAMA* 176, 50–51 (1961).

p.48   'Most notably, the immunologist David Strachan published his
        "clean hypothesis" in 1989, and this has since formed a guid-
        ing principle in applied research.' Strachan, D. P. Family size,
        infection and atopy: the first decade of the 'hygiene hypothesis'.
        Thorax 55, S2–S10 (2000).

3: SKIN AND BONES

p.54   'In total, the hospital cared for twenty-eight patients, many
        benefiting from the breakthrough "spray-on skin" devel-
        oped by the pioneering surgeon, Fiona Wood.' Wood, F.
        M., Stoner, M. L., Fowler, B. V. & Fear, M. W. The use of a
        non-cultured autologous cell suspension and Integra dermal
        regeneration template to repair full-thickness skin wounds
        in a porcine model: a one-step process. *Burns* 33, 693–700
        (2007).

p.57   'Wipe this habitat clean with disinfectant and just twelve hours
        later your exact microbial fingerprint will respawn as if using
        a time machine.' Fierer, N. *et al.* Forensic identification using
        skin bacterial communities. *Proc. Natl. Acad. Sci. U.S.A.* 107,
        6477–6481 (2010).

p.61   'This viewpoint is supported by neurocognitive evidence under-
        pinning Sam Harris' description of "the illusion of free will".'
        Harris, S. *Free Will.* (Simon & Schuster, 2012).

p.61   'Functional MRI studies, scanning areas of the brain involved
        in cognition, now show that subconscious processes prede-
        termine our choices long before we are even aware of "us"

making a decision.' Hallett, M. Volitional control of movement: the physiology of free will. *Clin Neurophysiol* 118, 1179–1192 (2007).

p.64 'With the development of machines such as IBM's supercomputer Watson, even this human integration based on knowledge and experience can be replicated.' Goetz, L. H. & Schork, N. J. Personalized medicine: motivation, challenges, and progress. *Fertil. Steril.* 109, 952–963 (2018).

p.66 '... the first weekend of March saw sixteen weather-related deaths as the heaviest snowfall in more than thirty-five years was dumped on an ill-prepared UK.' https://en.wikipedia.org/wiki/2018_Great_Britain_and_Ireland_cold_wave

p.66 '... one of the busiest periods for critical care services ever described, with my ICU swelling to over 170 per cent of its funded capacity.' Campbell, D. NHS intensive care units sending patients elsewhere due to lack of beds. *The Guardian* (2018).

p.67 '"When no longer able to change a situation, we are challenged to change ourselves."' Frankl, V. E. (2006). *Man's Search for Meaning.* Boston: Beacon Press.

p.68 '... talk about how business management methods can solve the woes of a hospital in crisis.' Westwood, N. *Going Lean in the NHS.* NHS England (2007).

p.72 'Globally, over 3,000 people die every day from road traffic collisions, that is 1.3 million deaths per year.' WHO. *Road traffic injuries.* World Health Organization (2018).

p.72 'However, the same cannot be said of low- and middle-income countries where – despite having only half of the world's vehicles – more than 90 per cent of all road fatalities occur.' These data all come from the reference provided above.

p.73 'The evolution of a blood-transfusion service was one of the most significant medical outcomes of the First World War.' Giangrande, P. L. F. The history of blood transfusion. *Br J Haematol* 110, 758–767 (2000).

4: THE HEART

p.78   'It was the first time she had ever called him by his first name.' So as to maintain anonymity, I have not used his name. A stickler for the facts (thankfully), The Judge didn't want me to embellish this part of his story by simply making up an imaginary name.

p.79   '. . . a key factor in what is known as the chain of survival.' Rao, P. & Kern, K. B. Improving Community Survival Rates from Out-of-Hospital Cardiac Arrest. *Curr Cardiol Rev* 14, 79–84 (2018).

p.79   'Every year, 30,000 people in the UK will suddenly collapse to the ground having suffered a cardiac arrest.' Perkins, G. D. & Brace-McDonnell, S. J. The UK Out of Hospital Cardiac Arrest Outcome (OHCAO) project. *BMJ Open* 5, e008736 (2015).

p.79   'Of these twenty, two will eventually return home to a relatively normal life.' Perkins, G. D. *et al.* A Randomized Trial of Epinephrine in Out-of-Hospital Cardiac Arrest. *N Engl J Med* 379, 711–721 (2018).

p.80   '. . . these have assumed a special place in the public consciousness even though CPR is often less effective than other optional therapies.' O'Brien, H. *et al.* Do-not-attempt-resuscitation (DNAR) orders: understanding and interpretation of their use in the hospitalised patient in Ireland. A brief report. *J Med Ethics* 44, 201–203 (2018).

p.81   'Providing a conduit for breath is the most ancient component of CPR, as revealed by stories in the Babylonian Talmud where a lamb with an injury to the neck was rescued by making a hole in the windpipe and inserting a hollow reed.' Rodkinson, M. L. *The Babylonian Talmud, Book 1 (Vols I and II)* (Pinnacle Press, 2017).

p.81   '. . . objects as diverse as ballpoint pens and drinking straws having been used to save lives.' Onrubia, X., Frova, G. & Sorbello, M. Front of neck access to the airway: A narrative review. *Trends in Anaesthesia and Critical Care* 22, 45–55 (2018).

p.81   'Advances in airway control continued when the Dutch Humane Society, founded in 1768 to help drowning victims, recommended using bizarre practices including rolling patients upside down in a barrel after water submersion.' Lee, R. V. Cardiopulmonary resuscitation in the eighteenth century. A historical perspective on present practice. *J Hist Med Allied Sci* 27, 418–433 (1972).

p.81 'The use of inflatable bags attached to oxygen improved upon the recommended technique of inserting a fire-bellows into people's nostrils and anus in the 1500s, hence the term "blowing smoke up one's arse".' Ball, C. M. & Featherstone, P. J. Early resuscitation practices. *Anaesth Intensive Care* 44, 3–4 (2016).

p.82 '. . . he resuscitated the coal miner James Blair by using mouth-to-mouth rescue breathing.' Trubuhovich, R. V. History of Mouth-to-Mouth Rescue Breathing. Part 1. *Crit Care Resusc* 7, 257 (2005).

p.82 'This comedic practice features in Arthur Conan Doyle's "The Adventure of the Stockbroker's Clerk" where, after Holmes discovers a business owner hanging by the neck from his braces, Watson successfully performs the chest-pressure arm-lift, saving the man's life.' Doyle, A. C. *The Memoirs of Sherlock Holmes (illustrated)* (Clap Publishing, LLC., 2018).

p.83 'This followed extensive work on resuscitation by Austrian doctor, Peter Safar, and an American, Dr James Elam.' Ball, C. M. & Featherstone, P. J. *op cit.*

p.84 '. . . from an abnormal heart rhythm after receiving small electric shocks.' Kouwenhoven, W. B., Langworthy, O. R., Singewald, M. L. & Knickerbocker, G. G. Medical Evaluation of Man Working in AC Electric Fields. *IEEE Transactions on Power Apparatus and Systems* PAS-86, 506–511 (1967).

p.84 'These AEDs can even be delivered by drones in remote areas, allowing lives to be saved where the delay waiting for an ambulance to arrive would otherwise prove fatal.' Boutilier, J. J. *et al.* Optimizing a Drone Network to Deliver Automated External Defibrillators. *Circulation* 135, 2454–2465 (2017).

p.85 'The lengths to which we will go may even involve performing life-saving open-heart surgery at the side of the road, as one of my medical school colleagues in the Welsh air ambulance service did in 2017.' Boutilier, J. J. *et al.* National Award for Rare Life-Saving Medical Procedure. *Circulation* 135, 2466–2469 (2017).

p.85   'French medical services have even put a patient having a cardiac arrest onto a portable heart-bypass machine in the middle of the Louvre in Paris while the *Mona Lisa* silently looked on.' Lamhaut, L. *et al.* Extracorporeal Cardiopulmonary Resuscitation (ECPR) in the Prehospital Setting: An Illustrative Case of ECPR Performed in the Louvre Museum. *Prehosp Emerg Care* 21, 386–389 (2017).

p.86   'My palliative care colleague, Dr Mark Taubert, has advanced this public discussion in a remarkable way through both his "Talk CPR" initiative which encourages conversation about resuscitation for people affected by life-limiting illnesses ...' Read more about this at http://talkcpr.com.

p.86   '... and his open letter published in the *British Medical Journal* in the wake of David Bowie's death, thanking the singer for helping others come to terms with death.' Vincent, A. Watch Jarvis Cocker read a letter to David Bowie: 'We wondered whether anyone was holding your hand'. *Daily Telegraph* (2016).

p.87   'If bystander CPR was performed consistently following cardiac arrest, on any given day thousands more lives could be saved.' Lindner, T. W., Søreide, E., Nilsen, O. B., Torunn, M. W. & Lossius, H. M. Good outcome in every fourth resuscitation attempt is achievable – an Utstein template report from the Stavanger region. *Resuscitation* 82, 1508–1513 (2011).

p.91   '(This was a good thing as it showed that the force of the CPR was sufficient to allow blood to get to his brain.)' Hellevuo, H. *et al.* Deeper chest compression – more complications for cardiac arrest patients? *Resuscitation* 84, 760–765 (2013).

p.92   'We are currently conducting a large international clinical trial to help answer this very question.' Nielsen, N. *et al.* Targeted Temperature Management at 33°C versus 36°C after Cardiac Arrest. *N Engl J Med.* Massachusetts Medical Society; 2013 Dec 5;369(23):2197–206.

p.94   'Nearly every mammal on earth, big and small, maintains a remarkable relationship between its average life expectancy and heart rate.' Levine, H. J. Rest heart rate and life expectancy. *J. Am. Coll. Cardiol.* 30, 1104–1106 (1997).

p.95   '... the blue whale's plod of just six heartbeats per minute is linked with an average life expectancy of over a hundred years.' Ponganis, P. J. & Kooyman, G. L. Heart Rate and Electrocardiogram Characteristics of a Young California Gray Whale (*Eschrichtius robustus*) *Marine Mammal Science* 15, 1198–1207 (2006).

p.95   'People living at home with even relatively mild forms of heart failure have a shorter life expectancy than some patients with cancer.' Stewart, S., MacIntyre, K., Hole, D. J., Capewell, S. & McMurray, J. J. More 'malignant' than cancer? Five-year survival following a first admission for heart failure. *Eur. J. Heart Fail.* 3, 315–322 (2001).

p.95   'During a typical six-minute period of sexual intercourse ('typical' hides a wide variation, of course), your heart increases its number of beats from 400 to over 1,000.' Corty, E. W. & Guardiani, J. M. Canadian and American sex therapists' perceptions of normal and abnormal ejaculatory latencies: how long should intercourse last? *J Sex Med* 5, 1251–1256 (2008).

p.96   '... these physiological changes start developing from just five weeks into pregnancy.' Hunter, S. & Robson, S. C. Adaptation of the maternal heart in pregnancy. *Br Heart J* 68, 540–543 (1992).

p.97   'Chronic health conditions, including high blood pressure, obesity, smoking and ischemic heart disease, account for over 90 per cent of cases of heart failure.' Piepoli, M. F. *et al.* Main messages for primary care from the 2016 European Guidelines on cardiovascular disease prevention in clinical practice. *Eur J Gen Pract* 24, 51–56 (2018).

p.99   ' ... throughout the course of mammalian evolution.' Chuong, E. B. Retroviruses facilitate the rapid evolution of the mammalian placenta. *Bioessays* 35, 853–861 (2013).

p.102   'Medicine has had a long-standing fascination with the heart since William Harvey first described it as "the circuit of the blood" in 1628.' Harvey, W. & Bowie, A. *On the Motion of the Heart and Blood in Animals, Volumes 1–3.* (Palala Press, 2018).

p.102   '. . . its function replaced by two implanted mechanical pumps.' Pirk, J. *et al.* Total artificial heart support with two continuous-flow ventricular assist devices in a patient with an infiltrating cardiac sarcoma. *ASAIO J.* 59, 178–180 (2013).

p.103   '. . . the average wait on a transplant list is nearly three years.' NHSBT. *Organ Donation and Transplantation Activity Report 2017/18. NHSBT* (2018).

p.103   '(In fact, this was the first heart transplant performed in humans.)' Cooper, D. K. C. A brief history of cross-species organ transplantation. *Proc (Bayl Univ Med Cent)* 25, 49–57 (2012).

p.103   'However, most experts believe that this is still two to five years away and likely to start with kidney transplants between genetically engineered pigs and humans.' Servick, K. Xenotransplant advances may prompt human trials. *Science* 357, 1338–1338 (2017).

p.104   '. . . an eighteen-year-old woman survived after having a hole in her heart closed using an "Iron Heart" machine'. Passaroni, A. C., Silva, M. A. de M. & Yoshida, W. B. Cardiopulmonary bypass: development of John Gibbon's heart-lung machine. *Rev Bras Cir Cardiovasc* 30, 235–245 (2015).

5: THE LUNGS

p.108   '"I have seen many a man turn his gold into smoke, but you are the first who has turned smoke into gold."' S.A. Bent, comp. Familiar Short Sayings of Great Men. 1887.

p.109   'It causes nearly 8 million deaths annually, 10 per cent of which are due to second-hand smoke.' National Center for Chronic Disease Prevention and Health Promotion (US) Office on Smoking and Health. The Health Consequences of Smoking – 50 Years of Progress: A Report of the Surgeon General. (2014).

p.109   'One in five deaths are tobacco-related, with smokers dying ten years earlier than non-smokers on average.' *ibid.*

p.109   'Nearly 15 per cent of these substances are tobacco-related, compared with 9 per cent from alcohol and 5 per cent from illicit drugs.' Jolivot, P.-A. *et al.* An observational study of adult admissions to a medical ICU due to adverse drug events. *Ann Intensive Care* 6, 9 (2016).

p.110   '... the map that the English physician, John Snow, drew 160 years ago when examining the cause of this deadly cholera outbreak contained something far more telling.' Hajna, S., Buckeridge, D. L. & Hanley, J. A. Substantiating the impact of John Snow's contributions using data deleted during the 1936 reprinting of his original essay On the Mode of Communication of Cholera. *Int. J. Epidemiol.* 44, 1794–1799 (2015).

p.117   'In COPD, this type of lung support can prevent the need for a life-support machine and improve a patient's chances of survival.' Quinnell, T. G., Pilsworth, S., Shneerson, J. M. & Smith, I. E. Prolonged invasive ventilation following acute ventilatory failure in COPD: weaning results, survival, and the role of noninvasive ventilation. *Chest* 129, 133–139 (2006).

p.119   '... caffeine is a naturally occurring phosphodiesterase inhibitor that can be used in rural locations without medical facilities to help treat tight lungs.' Johnson, C. & Winser, S. *Oxford Handbook of Expedition and Wilderness Medicine.* (Oxford University Press, USA, 2015).

p.124   '... promoting randomised control trials (RCTs) as the best method to conduct medical research.' Hill, G. B. Archie Cochrane and his legacy. An internal challenge to physicians' autonomy? *Journal of clinical epidemiology* 53, 1189–1192 (2000).

p.125   '... 90 per cent of what I do will not be based upon this level of evidence.' Zhang, Z., Hong, Y. & Liu, N. Scientific evidence underlying the recommendations of critical care clinical practice guidelines: a lack of high level evidence. *Intensive Care Med* 44, 1189–1191 (2018).

p.125   'If the stethoscope were to be invented today, it would most likely not meet the current standards needed for approval of a medical device.' Hubmayr, R. D. The times are a-changin': should we hang up the stethoscope? *Anesthesiology* 100, 1–2 (2004).

p.127   'The "Winter Crisis" is now simply "The Crisis" as countless newspaper articles report.' Marsh, S. NHS is facing year-round crisis, says British Medical Association (2018).

References

p.127   '... as few as one in ten of our treatments are based on the highest quality evidence.' Zhang, Z., Hong, Y. & Liu, N. Scientific evidence underlying the recommendations of critical care clinical practice guidelines: a lack of high level evidence. *op cit.*

p.128   'If you are treated in a hospital that does research, you too are more likely to live than to die.' Ozdemir, B. A. *et al.* Research activity and the association with mortality. *PloS ONE* 10, e0118253 (2015).

p.129   '... it was the hard graft of research teams producing a safe, effective vaccine ...' Stefanelli, P. & Rezza, G. Impact of vaccination on meningococcal epidemiology. *Hum Vaccin Immunother* 12, 1051–1055 (2016).

p.129   'For example, a major international clinical trial in our unit examines the best temperature to use when cooling patients like The Judge following a cardiac arrest.' Nielsen, N. *et al. op cit.*

p.131   'Trials using this approach have already had a real, tangible and prolonged positive effect on the care of the sickest patients all around the world.' CRASH-2 trial collaborators *et al.* Effects of tranexamic acid on death, vascular occlusive events, and blood transfusion in trauma patients with significant haemorrhage (CRASH-2): a randomised, placebo-controlled trial. *The Lancet* 376, 23–32 (2010).

p.131   'It is estimated that over half of all studies are never completed and data from one-third of trials not published.' Goldacre, B. Are clinical trial data shared sufficiently today? No. *BMJ* 347, f1880–f1880 (2013).

p.131   'Of those that are, only half are read by more than just two people.' Smith, R. The trouble with medical journals. *J R Soc Med* 99, 115–119 (2006).

p.131   '... that the entire medical journal industry should be disbanded.' Smith, R. *ibid.*

p.132   'The late Dr Kate Granger was an inspirational British doctor who recognised this fact.' Granger, K. Healthcare staff must properly introduce themselves to patients. *BMJ* 347, f5833–f5833 (2013).

p.133   '... that around 3,000 patients live in their own homes, needing a ventilator, in the UK.' Lloyd-Owen, S. J. *et al.* Patterns of home mechanical ventilation use in Europe: results from the Eurovent survey. *Eur. Respir. J.* 25, 1025–1031 (2005).

p.134   'Muscle wasting occurs just hours into a period of critical illness ...' Puthucheary, Z. A. *et al.* Acute skeletal muscle wasting in critical illness. *JAMA* 310, 1591–1600 (2013).

p.137   'You are almost twice as likely to survive today from sepsis – the main reason for admissions to the ICU – than fifteen years ago.' Stevenson, E. K., Rubenstein, A. R., Radin, G. T., Wiener, R. S. & Walkey, A. J. Two Decades of Mortality Trends Among Patients With Severe Sepsis. *Critical Care Medicine* 42, 625–631 (2014).

p.137   'The chances of you getting home following a cardiac arrest in the community are 25 per cent better today than just a decade ago.' Daya, M. R. *et al.* Out-of-hospital cardiac arrest survival improving over time: Results from the Resuscitation Outcomes Consortium (ROC). *Resuscitation* 91, 108–115 (2015).

6: THE BRAIN

p.140   'This scale was developed by Professor Jennett and his trainee Dr Teasdale (now Sir Graham) in 1974 ...' Teasdale, G. & Jennett, B. Assessment of coma and impaired consciousness. A practical scale. *The Lancet* 2, 81–84 (1974).

p.143   'When propofol was used by Dr Conrad Murray, the side effects of this white, milky emulsion led to the death of the world's greatest pop star.' http://i2.cdn.turner.com/cnn/2010/images/02/09/mj_autopsy.pdf.

p.143   'Instead, he left Jackson alone while he visited the toilet.' https://www.omicsonline.org/the-michael-jackson-autopsy-insights-provided-by-a-forensic-anesthesiologist-2157-7145.1000138.pdf.

p.144   'You are far more likely to get hit by a bus on your way to hospital than to experience this rare phenomenon after arriving.' Walker, E. M. K., Bell, M., Cook, T. M., Grocott, M. P. W. & Moonesinghe, S. R. Patient reported outcome of adult perioperative anaesthesia in the United Kingdom: a cross-sectional observational study. *British Journal of Anaesthesia* 117, 758–766r (2016).

p.150   'The book *Blink* by my hero, Malcolm Gladwell ...' Gladwell, M. *Blink* (Hachette UK, 2007).

p.150   '(This was based on the work of Nobel Prize winner Daniel Kahneman and his late colleague Amos Tversky.)' Kahneman, D. & Tversky, A. On the reality of cognitive illusions. *Psychol Rev* 103, 582–91– discussion 592–6 (1996).

p.152   'Later, as a fighter pilot in the Second World War, he came close to death after landing his Gloster Gladiator biplane hard in the Egyptian desert and breaking his nose, fracturing his skull and being knocked unconscious.' *Storyteller: The Life of Roald Dahl*, Donald Sturrock (William Collins, 2016).

p.152   'There was no effective vaccination, so Dahl acquired a single dose of "gamma globulin" for his son from the head of the Lister Institute of Preventive Medicine, who was married to Dahl's half-sister and who agreed to import this gamma globulin from America.' *ibid.*

p.152   'Olivia had died because the measles virus had spread to her brain, inflaming the delicate, tissue-thin linings and causing encephalitis.' *ibid.*

p.153   'Public health authorities still use this letter in publicity campaigns today.' Baddeley, A. Roald Dahl's measles warning inspires parents. *Daily Telegraph* (2015).

p.154   'It is tragic that 2013–18 has seen the rate of measles infections rise by over 300 per cent across Europe ...' Boseley, S. WHO warns over measles immunisation rates as cases rise 300% across Europe. *The Guardian* (2018).

p.154   '"Surely one hour a day is not enough. What in the world are you going to teach a child if she only goes to school for an hour a day?"' Sturrock, D. *op cit.*

p.155   '"Slowly, insidiously and quite relentlessly" ...' *Roald Dahl's Marvellous Medicine*, Tom Solomon, Liverpool University Press, 2016.

p.155   '... a book that led to the formation of the Stroke Association.' Neal, P. *As I Am* (Simon & Schuster, 2011).

p.156   'The fantastic book *Why We Sleep*, by the American neuroscientist Matthew Walker, beautifully translates these costs into human terms while explaining the science behind our essential slumber.' Walker, M. P. (2017). *Why We Sleep: Unlocking the power of sleep and dreams* (First Scribner hardcover edition.). New York: Scribner.

p.157   'Night-shift workers in Denmark who developed breast cancer after years of working night shifts have even received compensation based on this evidence.' Danish night shift workers with breast cancer awarded compensation. *BMJ* 2009;338:b1152.

p.157   'She would not finish these and instead died tragically on 17 September 2011 on Scotland's busiest motorway as she fell asleep at the wheel of her car.' Facts from a discussion with her dad, Brian Connelly and from Worked to death – exhausted young doctor veers off road and dies after gruelling nightshift, *Daily Record*, Stephen Stewart, 16/10/2011.

p.157   '... my chances of having a crash are nearly twelve times higher than someone who has slept for seven hours.' Liu, S.-Y., Perez, M. A. & Lau, N. The impact of sleep disorders on driving safety – findings from the Second Strategic Highway Research Program naturalistic driving study. *Sleep* 41, 298 (2018).

p.160   '... up to 80 per cent of intensive care patients will experience it at some point.' Ouimet, S., Kavanagh, B. P., Gottfried, S. B. & Skrobik, Y. Incidence, risk factors and consequences of ICU delirium. *Intensive Care Med* 33, 66–73 (2007).

p.164   'Transfusing blood to achieve a normal level of haemoglobin has been shown to cause more deaths.' Chohan, S. S., McArdle, F., McClelland, D. B. L., Mackenzie, S. J. & Walsh, T. S. Red cell transfusion practice following the transfusion requirements in critical care (TRICC) study: prospective observational cohort study in a large UK intensive care unit. *Vox Sang.* 84, 211–218 (2003).

p.164   'Giving high amounts of oxygen to people with bad lungs may cause more deaths.' Panwar, R. *et al.* Conservative versus Liberal Oxygenation Targets for Mechanically Ventilated Patients. A Pilot Multicenter Randomized Controlled Trial. *American Journal of Respiratory and Critical Care Medicine* 193, 43–51 (2016).

p.164   '... a decompressive craniectomy does produce more survivors, but with an increased likelihood of severe, profound disability overall.' Cooper, D. J. *et al.* Decompressive Craniectomy in Diffuse Traumatic Brain Injury. *N Engl J Med* 364, 1493–1502 (2011).

p.166   '... gel-like material produced by bacteria (a biofilm) forms around the plastic of breathing tubes.' Sands, K. M. *et al.* Respiratory pathogen colonization of dental plaque, the lower airways, and endotracheal tube biofilms during mechanical ventilation. *J Crit Care* 37, 30–37 (2017).

7: THE GUTS

p.175   'Along with tobacco, alcohol is by far the most dangerous recreational drug that we encounter in intensive care.' Secombe, P. J. & Stewart, P. C. The impact of alcohol-related admissions on resource use in critically ill patients from 2009 to 2015: an observational study. *Anaesth Intensive Care* 46, 58–66 (2018).

p.178   'While, globally, infections of the liver are the most common reasons for its failure, it is unsurprising that alcohol consumption is the leading cause in the Western world.' Bernal, W., Auzinger, G., Dhawan, A. & Wendon, J. Acute liver failure. *The Lancet* 376, 190–201 (2010).

p.178   'In over one-third of patients with liver failure, alcohol is the prime cause ...' *ibid.*

p.178   '... one in two liver transplants occur as a result of liver failure from alcohol misuse.' European Liver Transplant Registry. Available at: http://www.eltr.org/Specific-results-by-disease.html (Accessed: 1 October 2018).

p.178   '... alcoholic liver disease has been estimated to kill more people than diabetes and road collisions combined.' Facts About Liver Disease – British Liver Trust.

p.183   '... they will lose as much as 20 per cent of their muscle mass within three days.' Puthucheary, Z. A. *et al.* Acute skeletal muscle wasting in critical illness. *JAMA* 310, 1591–1600 (2013).

p.183   'The mechanical work performed by our breathing machines also thins the diaphragm after just twenty-four hours of use.' Facts About Liver Disease, *op cit.*

p.183 'Occasionally body scanners designed for zoo animals have been considered to help get a diagnosis in humans.' Hawley, P. C. & Hawley, M. P. Difficulties in diagnosing pulmonary embolism in the obese patient: A literature review. *Vasc Med* 16, 444–451 (2011).

p.184 'The misleading campaigns offering "low-fat" alternatives may have conversely led to escalating levels of obesity . . .' Ludwig, D. S. *Always Hungry?* (Hachette UK, 2016).

p.184 '. . . due to replacement of fat content . . .' Bazzano, L. A. *et al.* Effects of low-carbohydrate and low-fat diets: a randomized trial. *Ann. Intern. Med.* 161, 309–318 (2014).

p.184 '. . . with refined sugars.' Siri-Tarino, P. W., Sun, Q., Hu, F. B. & Krauss, R. M. Meta-analysis of prospective cohort studies evaluating the association of saturated fat with cardiovascular disease. *Am. J. Clin. Nutr.* 91, 535–546 (2010).

p.186 'Named after New York physician Dr Burrill Crohn in 1932 . . .' Geller, S. A. in *Encyclopedia of Pathology* (ed. van Krieken, J. H. J. M.) 1–4 (Springer International Publishing, 2016).

p.186 '. . . likely reasons include environmental infections, genetic predisposition and lifestyle choices.' Sartor, R. B. Mechanisms of disease: pathogenesis of Crohn's disease and ulcerative colitis. *Nat Clin Pract Gastroenterol Hepatol* 3, 390–407 (2006).

p.188 'A laparotomy is the most common operation to result in critical illness.' Saunders, D. I. *et al.* Variations in mortality after emergency laparotomy: the first report of the UK Emergency Laparotomy Network. *British Journal of Anaesthesia* 109, 368–375 (2012).

p.191 'Total parenteral nutrition (TPN) was first used in 1969 by doctors treating newborns with bowel cancer.' Dudrick, S. J. History of parenteral nutrition. *J Am Coll Nutr* 28, 243–251 (2009).

p.194 'Today, your chances of surviving after a laparotomy are double those of forty years ago.' Palmberg, S. & Hirsjärvi, E. Mortality in Geriatric Surgery. *Gerontology* 25, 103–112 (1979).

p.194 'We have learnt lessons from space exploration on how to nourish and maintain the body's muscles when under extreme stress.' Hides, J. *et al*. Parallels between astronauts and terrestrial patients – Taking physiotherapy rehabilitation 'To infinity and beyond'. *Musculoskelet Sci Pract* 27 Suppl 1, S32–S37 (2017).

p.194   'Machines that replace the functions of the liver ...' Nicolas, C. T. *et al*. Concise Review: Liver Regenerative Medicine: From Hepatocyte Transplantation to Bioartificial Livers and Bioengineered Grafts. *Stem Cells* 35, 42–50 (2017).

p.194   '... and pancreas ...' Breton, M. *et al*. Fully integrated artificial pancreas in type 1 diabetes: modular closed-loop glucose control maintains near normoglycemia. *Diabetes* 61, 2230–2237 (2012).

8: THE BLOOD

p.195   'Carl Sagan, one of the most celebrated scientists of the last 100 years, famously said, "We are made of star-stuff."' *The Cosmic Connection: An Extraterrestrial Perspective*. Carl Sagan. Doubleday, New York, 1973.

p.197   '... I would be twice as likely to discover a blood clot after a long-haul flight.' Schwarz, T. *et al*. Venous thrombosis after long-haul flights. *Arch. Intern. Med.* 163, 2759–2764 (2003).

p.197   'It is no wonder that his friends described him as the "pope of medicine"'. Silver, G. A. Virchow, the heroic model in medicine: health policy by accolade. *American Journal of Public Health* 77, 82–88 (American Public Health Association, 1987).

p.198   'There are few evidence-based treatments that have been shown definitively to cure disease in critical care ...' Zhang, Z., Hong, Y. & Liu, N. Scientific evidence underlying the recommendations of critical care clinical practice guidelines: a lack of high level evidence. *op cit*.

p.198   '... nearly one-third of critically ill patients will develop blood clots.' Geerts, W. & Selby, R. Prevention of venous thromboembolism in the ICU. *Chest* 124, 357S–363S (2003).

p.200   'Producing medical images using ultrasound was first introduced in 1942 by Austrian Dr Karl Theodore ...' Shampo, M. A. & Kyle, R. A. Karl Theodore Dussik – pioneer in ultrasound. *Mayo Clinic Proceedings* 70, (1995).

p.201   'The practical applications were significantly improved by the Scottish professor Ian Donald in the 1950s after he saw it being used in the shipyards of Glasgow to identify flaws in metal seams.' Kurjak, A. Ultrasound scanning – Prof. Ian Donald (1910-1987). *European Journal of Obstetrics, Gynecology, and Reproductive Biology* 90, 187–189 (2000).

p.201   '... he used these "metal flaw detector" techniques to instead find human flaws.' A brief history of musculoskeletal ultrasound: 'From bats and ships to babies and hips'. Kane, D. *et al*. *Rheumatology* 2004 Jul;43(7):931-3.

p.205   'The stress placed on the abdominal aorta, even when we are healthy, is high.' Oyre, S., Pedersen, E. M., Ringgaard, S., Boesiger, P. & Paaske, W. P. In vivo wall shear stress measured by magnetic resonance velocity mapping in the normal human abdominal aorta. *Eur J Vasc Endovasc Surg* 13, 263–271 (1997).

p.206   'He discovered early links between smoking and lung cancer, performed one of the world's first heart-bypass surgeries and introduced operations still essential to save lives in my hospital today.' Oransky, I. Michael E DeBakey. *The Lancet* 372, 530 (2008).

p.206   'He even trialled the first mechanical heart device that is now fast becoming a reasonable alternative to a heart transplant for some patients.' Mancini, D. & Colombo, P. C. Left Ventricular Assist Devices. *J. Am. Coll. Cardiol.* 65, 2542–2555 (2015).

p.212   'The success of this and other screening programmes led to its expansion nationwide ...' Logan, A. J. & Bourantas, N. I. Mortality from ruptured abdominal aortic aneurysm in Wales. *Br J Surg* 87, 966–967 (2000).

p.212   '... and is estimated to have halved the number of deaths from ruptured aneurysms.' Ashton, H. A. *et al*. The Multicentre Aneurysm Screening Study (MASS) into the effect of abdominal aortic aneurysm screening on mortality in men: a randomised controlled trial. *The Lancet* 360, 1531–1539 (2002).

9: THE SOUL

p.213 'Overall, one in five patients admitted will die ...' Prin, M. & Wunsch, H. International comparisons of intensive care: informing outcomes and improving standards. *Current Opinion in Critical Care* 18, 700–706 (2012).

p.214 'A total of twenty young people, with their lives ahead of them, died through hanging in just three months ...' Jones, P. *et al.* Identifying probable suicide clusters in Wales using national mortality data. *PLoS ONE* 8, e71713 (2013).

p.214 'Today, one in three patients with terminal cancer will die following an intensive care admission.' Cardona-Morrell, M. *et al.* Non-beneficial treatments in hospital at the end of life: a systematic review on extent of the problem. *Int J Qual Health Care* 28, 456–469 (2016).

p.214 'This has been shown to cause more pain and more distress and to incur more costs than effective palliative care.' Dalal, S. & Bruera, E. End-of-Life Care Matters: Palliative Cancer Care Results in Better Care and Lower Costs. *Oncologist* 22, 361–368 (2017).

pp.214–5 'Doctors are twice as likely as all other professions to kill themselves, with a staggering one in twenty-five doctors' deaths being attributable to suicide.' Hawton, K., Agerbo, E., Simkin, S., Platt, B. & Mellanby, R. J. Risk of suicide in medical and related occupational groups: a national study based on Danish case population-based registers. *J Affect Disord* 134, 320–326 (2011).

p.215 'This figure grows even greater for doctors facing patient complaints.' Hawton, K. Suicide in doctors while under fitness to practise investigation. *BMJ* 350, h813–h813 (2015).

p.215 'When I asked about her fascinating life, she encouraged me to buy a book she had written entitled *The Girl in the Spotty Dress*.' Stewart, P. & Clark, V. *The Girl in the Spotty Dress: Memories from the 1950s and the Photo That Changed My Life* (John Blake Publishing Ltd, 2016).

p.224 '"Death, perhaps uniquely among objects of our dread, instructs us how to live.'" Derren Brown, *Happy: Why More or Less Everything is Absolutely Fine*, Bantam Press.

p.225   '... to raise awareness of sepsis as the killer of more people every year than breast, lung and prostate cancer combined.' McPherson, D. *et al*. Sepsis-associated mortality in England: an analysis of multiple cause of death data from 2001 to 2010. *BMJ Open* 3, e002586 (2013).

p.226   '... a number of guidelines including that from the Academy of Medical Royal Colleges ...' Simpson, P. *et al*. A code of practice for the diagnosis and confirmation of death. *The Academy of Medical Royal Colleges* (2008).

ABOUT THE AUTHOR

Dr Matt Morgan is a consultant in intensive care medicine at the University Hospital of Wales, and an honorary senior research fellow at Cardiff University. He has worked in some of the largest British and Australasian hospitals and won prizes for research, including his PhD, which used artificial intelligence to solve complex medical problems. He is passionate about public engagement and has contributed to multiple scientific articles and books. He lives in Cardiff with his family.